To Maggie

Happy reading

Best Wishes from

Rosemary Laird

Covid Chronicles in Rhyme

Covid-19 pandemic recorded week by week in rhyming couplets

Rosemary Laird

First hardback edition

Book design by PublishingPush
All photographs are copyright © Rosemary Calvert

ISBN
978-1-80227-366-3 (paperback)
978-1-80227-367-0 (eBook)
978-1-80227-397-7 (hardback)

Covid Chronicles in Rhyme

Covid-19 pandemic recorded week by week in rhyming couplets

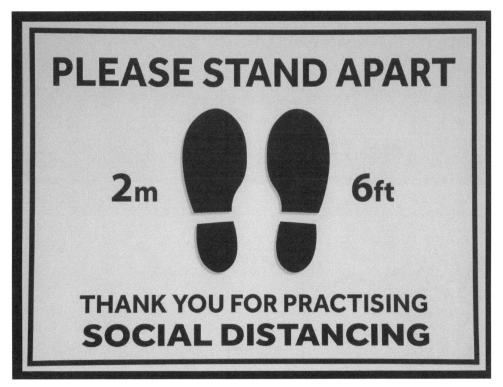

Rosemary Laird.

www.covid-chronicles-in-rhyme.com
(Professional photographer – Rosemary Calvert B.Ed. FRPS FRGS)
(www.rosemarycalvert.com)

Acknowledgements

BBC Radio 4 has been a wonderful source of information and inspiration during the 22 months of the Covid-19 Pandemic I've recorded here in 'Covid Chronicles in Rhyme'. Details of happenings, vaccines and drugs were gleaned from 'Today', the 'World at One' and 'PM programme'. Regular news updates on the hour helped to reinforce the news and daily BBC News on my iPad helped me to add and confirm detail. I would like to thank BBC Radio 4 for its first-class content and presentation.

The internet has served me well. I have no idea how many sites I should thank for just being there. I'm grateful for the existence of the internet and give thanks to the contributions that I've accessed for detailed information related to the Covid-19 pandemic. It is their contribution that has allowed me to provide accurate information in this book.

Contents

Introduction

On March 13th 2020, we were staying in the Swedish Ice Hotel celebrating my birthday. We'd had a normal flight out on 11th March but by the time we flew home on the 14th, the life we were accustomed to had evaporated. Stockholm airport was deserted, the huge corridors seeming to echo and assistants stood alone in the shops. The restaurants and airport lounges were closed and there was one food outlet. On the plane home, flight attendants cowered behind a curtain and there was no service.

Coronavirus had started to sweep across the world. I'm a photographer by profession but when I realised the seriousness of what was about to unfold, I felt moved to record events in words. A diary was the obvious choice but it seemed a rather unexciting way to create a record. Poetry, I felt, would bring an added interest and make my records a more compelling read in the future.

The weekly records in 'Covid Chronicles in Rhyme' start the day after lockdown. On Monday 23rd March 2020, Prime Minister Boris Johnson announced in a televised address that we must all stay at home. Only in exceptional circumstances could we leave our homes. Fortunately, food shopping came under this heading.

My poems at first reflect a light-hearted reaction to restrictions and risk but later they become more serious and an accurate weekly account with statistics and details of drugs and vaccines. Poetry takes second place as facts and statistics create what is sometimes a dark and depressing picture. The rhyming couplets remain and each weekly account, however grim, ends with a more optimistic or humorous verse.

Gardens are often mentioned in the poems. I love gardening and photograph my garden throughout the year. The poems are grouped by month and a seasonal garden photo heralds each month. I hope they will help paint a picture of the passing seasons as the Covid infection continues and the months pass. Illustrations also include a selection from the myriad of posters and signs which began to spring up everywhere to remind us of restrictions, indicate test sites and eventually direct us to vaccination centres.

When Covid-19 infections become routine and it's a disease we can live with, I hope 'Covid Chronicles in Rhyme' will endure and become a reminder of the difficult times we suffered and the wonder of the human resources it revealed.

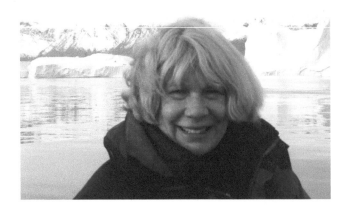

About the author

Rosemary was born Rosemary Phillips on 13 March 1945. She married and became Rosemary Calvert and then remarried and became Rosemary Laird. Her life has been varied, active and exciting.

Trained at Roehampton Froebel, she taught for 3 years before leaving to travel the world with her first husband who worked for an oil company. She turned her hand to whatever life had to offer from acting in Sarawak to being president of a camera club in Canada. Then after 28 years, she returned to the UK on her own.

Having discovered her photographs sold, she resolved to start a new life as a professional photographer. Sales grew and she signed up to 8 agencies who marketed her work. She now has 10,000 photos with Getty Images and reaches markets across the world. The 10 years she spent on her own were filled with photo trips to Antarctica, the Arctic and many other countries.

Rosemary was brought up in a family of 5 girls and, having also had a long happy marriage, she was used to sharing her life. So, after 10 years on her own, she turned to the internet to fill the gap. After 17 iffy internet dates, she found her man. Number 18 was a winner and in 2007 she married Angus Laird.

In 2020, 13 years later, the Pandemic struck. Rosemary felt it was time to put pen to paper and record a changing world where fear, sadness, compassion, inventiveness and triumph would all feature in excessive amounts.

A diary seemed the obvious way to record events as they unfolded but poetry seemed a more compelling way to chronicle this bizarre period in history. 'Covid Chronicles in Rhyme' was born and as it grew, it evolved. Rosemary hopes it will serve to remind readers of the totally shocking but sometimes wonderful times we all endured.

MARCH 2020 – JANUARY 2022

MARCH 2020

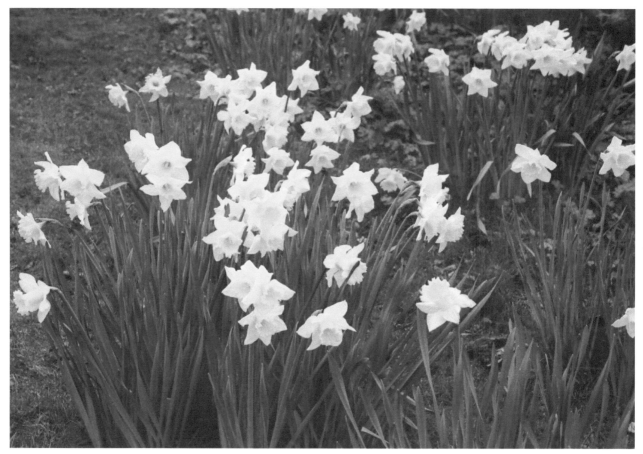

Daffodils blooming in the orchard.

Prime Minister Boris Johnson announced the first lockdown 23rd March 2020.

Week 1
24th March 2020

Covid-19 seems here to stay
And we must survive it in every way;

Cut our own hair, wash our hands,
Buy lots of loo rolls, amongst other plans.

Cancel the cruise, garage the car,
Buy tins of beans and stock up the bar.

Walk round the block two metres from you
And pick up the pills; what else can you do?

Not much, so it seems, no fun is allowed,
No touching, no kissing or joining the crowd.

But the garden invites us to work outside
To create beauty with love and swell with pride.

Over 70 we are and vulnerable too
But we'll give it our best and stay safe me and you.

APRIL 2020

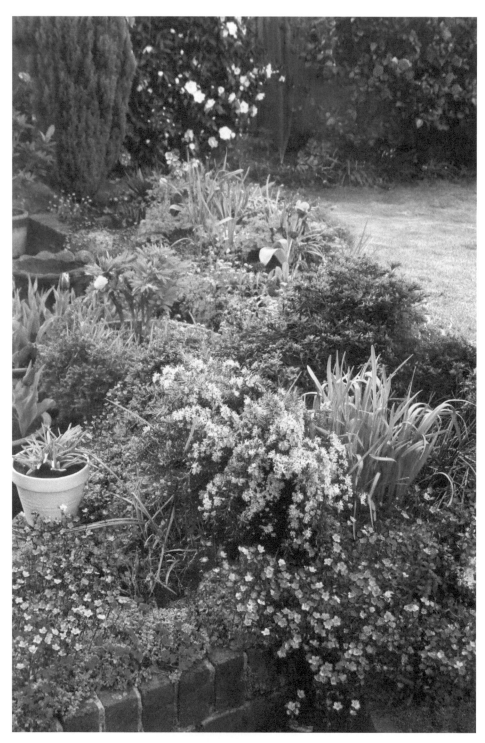

Frosty spring border

Week 2
April 4th 2020

Lockdown is nearly two weeks old
And most of us are doing exactly what we're told.

But still casualties rise and the virus with stealth is creeping,
Relentlessly each day, despite the Government's briefing.

One Nightingale hospital is open and ready
With five hundred beds, so progress is steady.

Testing will ramp up to a hundred thousand a day
And we will be cared for in every way.

Unless we are seventy-five plus, in a care home
Because if we are, then we're on our own.

Please don't phone for an ambulance because there are only a few
And much younger and fitter people are first in the queue.

Prince Charles and Matt Hancock have recovered we're told
But poor Boris is struggling to return to the fold.

Daffodils fade and hyacinths are bright
As each day we are filling until day becomes night.

For the garden is king and the sunshine is plenty
As we make our way through the year 2020.

Week 3
10ᵗʰ April 2020

An address from our monarch started this week.
She said 'We'll succeed', as we move to the peak.

Nearly 3 weeks have gone; review won't go as planned.
We're in for the long haul, still everything's banned.

As the pandemic progresses, we try to flatten the curve,
Save lives, protect the NHS and all carers that serve.

Lift our spirits, gargle with whisky, brandy or gin.
But there's no evidence it helps, it would just be a sin.

No flour to make cakes, but there's chocolate online.
So the cravings we feel can be quenched, pass the wine.

But alcohol is best used in hand wipes today.
Keep washing those hands, buy wet wipes on eBay.

Wipe the doorbell, the knocker and open the gate.
Save the delivery workers from an uncertain fate.

Concern changed to shock – Boris is in critical care.
The seriousness of the illness brought home, we declare.

But we're happy to say Boris is slowly improving.
Sitting up in his bed, he's with clinicians engaging.

We're ramping things up in these unprecedented times.
More PPE, CPAPs and ICUS, our language climbs.

We've furloughed our workers, social distanced our friends.
As the pandemic continues, here's to hoping it ends.

Hydroxychloroquine might help, but we need to know more.
Masks? Do we, or don't we? We're really not sure.

It's a time of uncertainty, lockdown, or is it lockup?
 If the over seventies get infected, they're right out of luck.

While some young see their friends by downloading Zoom,
Couples may create a new baby boom.

But lucky are those with gardens; with somewhere to go,
For sunbathing in parks isn't allowed, don't you know?

Tulips start to bloom, camellias, magnolias too.
Our gardens are precious, not just for the view.

We hear aeroplanes none, cars travel infrequently.
Bumblebees buzz and birds sing so sweetly.

Shopper's Guide for the Pandemic Paranoid

21th April 2020

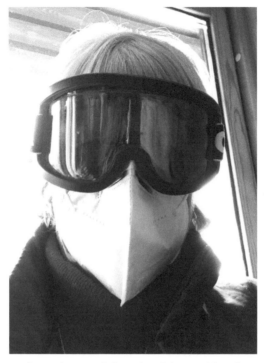

Author dressed for the bi-weekly shop

Log on at midnight, but you see you're already in a queue.
That's what is necessary here, so that's what you must do.

Watch the screen till one o'clock, of beauty sleep bereft.
You're through, hooray! But now you see no shopping slots are left.

With online food impossible, to the shops you must set out.
But Covid-19 awaits, of that there is no doubt.

Precautions then you must employ, wide aisles a good idea.
A Superstore would help keep to 2-metre rule, save the paranoia.

The old people's hour is early; set the alarm, it must be done.
Sacrifice more sleep, miss breakfast, get up before the sun.

Now before you leave there's lots to do, the shopping list but one.
Spray First Defence right up your nose, although it's not much fun.

Your mask must be N95 or FFP 2 – make doubly sure of that.
Alcohol wipes, 70% a must, no time to feed the cat.

Glasses are a good idea, sunglasses, ski goggles will do,
Just protect your eyes with something, it's really up to you.

Once there, a trolley you must seek, approach hand wipes in hand.
Wipe trolley handle well, it should be carefully planned.

Join the queue already formed marked out in airport style,
And make yourself comfortable, for you may be there a while.

The queue is clearly marked, you'll see, with sleeping trolleys used,
Wheels in the air and string between them, to keep you well amused.

Now clean your hands once more, you must remove the threat.
Put mask upon your face, but not too soon, it won't work if it gets wet.

Once in the store, you must avoid all shoppers that you meet.
Avoid them well for you must not get closer than six feet.

Two weeks' shopping you must buy, be careful what you choose.
What you forget you'll do without, so don't forget the booze.

Trolley parked and boot so full, return to learned refrain.
Wipe hands again, remove your mask and then wipe hands again.

Once home it's still not over; use First Defence once more,
Then gargle with salt water, you must be really sure.

Isolate shopping bags in shed, soapy wash or wipe food bought.
The coronavirus must be removed, Covid-19 must not be caught.

Your hands washed and wiped so many times, now dry and oh so sore.
They need hand cream, so rub it in, now that ends the shopping chore.

Totally exhausted, but hungry still, you really must be fed.
Then you are free, shopping complete, you can go back to bed.

Easter Special

April 12th 2020

Boris thanks the NHS for saving his life.
We thank them all for their work and their strife.

It's Easter Day, we have sunshine, skies a glorious blue,
But the beach is forbidden and our grandkids are too.

No church service to go to, may a virtual service suffice,
For churchgoers to celebrate the rising of Christ.

If the grandkids were here, we could Easter egg hunt.
We could picnic in the garden, choose the back or the front.

But we're here on our own and mustn't be blue.
We can paint faces on eggs and eat chocolate ones too.

We can sit in the garden, in the sunshine, do nothing,
For the pressure has gone to try to do something.

Has our life become tedious, what exciting things can we do?
Ah! The old vegetable leftovers, they'd make a fine stew.

'Alexa, country songs, please', we want to remember old times.
Or we could buy dangly earrings on Amazon Prime.

These extraordinary times change our thinking somehow.
 No eggs! Buy a chicken. No milk! Buy a cow.

But let's not be flippant, the world's in a mess.
Still, it's good to be silly, it helps with the stress.

Tulips still bloom, cherry blossom makes us prouder.
As we sit in the garden, the flutter of birds growing louder.

For over 70 we are and vulnerable too.
But we'll give it our best and stay safe me and you.

Week 4
April 17th 2020

STAY AT HOME is the message; stay behind the front door.
That's the way we embrace lockdown week number four.

Boris discharged, at Chequers recovering from his stay.
He thanks nurses who cared for him, says 'It could have gone either way'.

That's the good news. The bad news brings tears to our eyes.
The death toll tops 10,000, so many lost loved ones' lives.

A scientific advisor states the infection will gallop.
'The UK may be the worst affected country in Europe'.

Elderly in care homes dying, never hospitalized, untested.
PPE still lacking, they declare they're neglected.

By midweek news is changing, light is slowly creeping in.
A week starting so darkly filled with cautious optimism.

Hospital intake's reducing, the curve starting to flatten.
Lockdown is working and recovery starting to happen.

But lockdown will continue at least another three weeks.
Still, how can we expect freedom before Covid-19 peaks?

The care homes' plight has at last been addressed,
PPE promised, staff and residents will have the test.

Now it's Thursday again, time to clap at the door,
This week add a clap for Captain Tom Moore.

Ninety-nine years old before his 100th birthday has completed
One hundred laps of his garden. To NHS more than 18 million gifted.

Wonderful things are coming out of this extraordinary new normal.
People pulling together in both casual ways and formal.

'Lighthouse' mega-labs are up and running, getting on stream.
Antigen and antibody tests no longer a dream.

We must test everybody with symptoms and do it soon,
Then follow with testing those who may be immune.

Doctors are experimenting with drugs, drugs we have already.
We hope progress with recovery will improve and become steady.

New drugs we need fast and Remdesivir is in trial.
It's been used for Ebola but it may take a while.

A new vaccine is essential, researchers are doing their best.
It will take 12 to 18 months; there's little hope it could be less.

It's been sunny this week, a bit colder it's true.
Trees came to life, spring leaves a fresh green hue.

Our gardens are colourful, in sunshine they're bright.
Lucky to be alive are we, as dawn follows night.

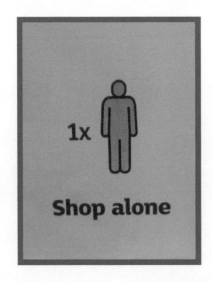
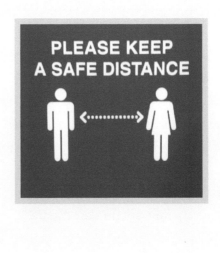

Pandemic posters - Shop alone and Keep a safe distance

Week 5
April 24th 2020

The Sunday papers launched week five with a message to alarm,
Over seventies must lockdown till end of 2021.

It wasn't true but all the same, the threat will long remain.
Our only hope's a new vaccine, to make coronavirus wane.

This week scientists in Oxford human vaccine trials began.
With just two volunteers they started but 5,000 is the plan.

Imperial College research goes on, we have great hopes there too.
Government funding supplied to both; we hope it sees them through.

Businessmen and academics a vaccine task force created.
They'll pull together developments until they're all collated.

Effective drugs we need, drugs to fulfil our expectation.
Dundee University test Brensocatib to fight lung inflammation.

With Remdesivir there were high hopes but trials proved inconclusive.
The stock markets fell across Europe, no longer are we to use it.

Queen's University in Belfast has massive drug trials on stream.
Dogs sniffing out the virus at airports is more than just a dream.

Test, track, trace and isolate, that's a good idea there is no doubt.
18,000 professional workers have been hired to carry the work out.

But amidst this good news, a squabble starts to brew.
Who did nothing and who said what to whom and was it true?

Has the horse now bolted and is the cat truly out of the bag?
Who took their eye off the ball, and did they allow time to lag?

We're certainly not out of the woods yet, too much fell upon deaf ears.
The light at the end of the tunnel but a faint glimmer, not enough to allay our fears.

Insufficient PPE supplied, such enormous quantities required.
400,000 gowns from Turkey delayed and home suppliers all ignored.

Lord Deighton to the rescue, PPE he will organize.
Front-line staff will be made safe, to include carers would be wise.

Relief we found this week from star-studded concert 'Together at home'.
With songs from Lady Gaga, Paul McCartney and the Rolling Stones.

'Big Night In' on Thursday featured stars and Royalty too
It raised 27 million pounds to boost charities anew.

Week five began with welcome rain; the water butts are full.
Plants and trees have been refreshed, our gardens bloom anew.

Now sunshine fills the greenhouse, the seedlings grow and thrive.
How thankful we are truly, thankful to be alive.

MAY 2020

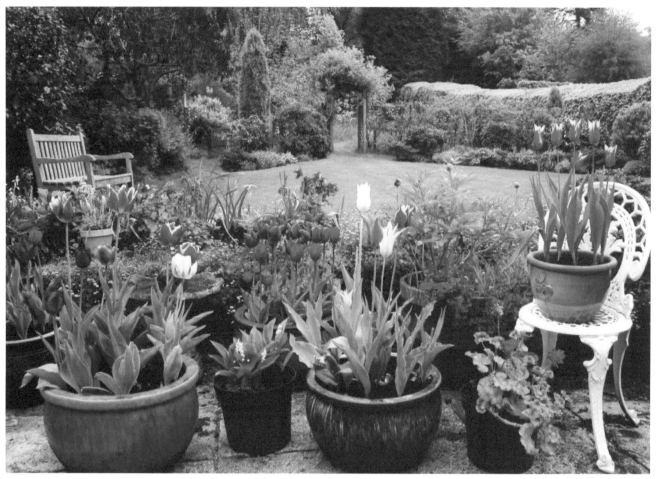

Late spring garden with pots of bright coloured tulips.

Week 6
May 1st 2020

Boris is back, it's week six and our leader is back in control.
Standing outside number 10 he maps out his ultimate goal.

'The tide has begun to turn,' he said, 'we're passing through the peak,
Lockdown is here to stay for now,' but then came a surprise midweek.

Congratulations to Boris and Carrie for the birth of their baby son.
Another resident for number 10 and broken nights for everyone.

A minute's silence on Tuesday for NHS staff, carers, key workers too,
85 NHS staff have died and 19 social carers. Far more than just a few

Captain Tom's 100th birthday on Thursday, a handwritten card from the queen.
Spitfire and Hurricane flypast, message from Boris Johnson on screen.

Now Tom's an honorary Colonel, raising over 32 million was great.
Number one in the charts with Michael Ball, now that's what he's achieved to date.

Goal of 100,000 tests has been achieved, 25,000 home testing kits sent out.
48 drive-through centres, 70 mobile units, success is no longer in doubt.

Testing is up, R rate is coming down, but it must stay below one before —
Lockdown is reconsidered, a second spike prevented, virus infection not allowed to soar.

Remdesivir is back in the news once more and the US results are encouraging.
It speeds up recovery of that they're sure. Their trials haven't come to nothing.

AstraZeneca will produce the vaccine if Oxford University trials are a success.
End of year it could be ready and then the spread of Covid-19 will become less.

Now the death rate is shocking. A third of those admitted to hospital have died.
Ethnic minorities, obese and aged worst affected, data has now been supplied.

Death in deprived areas is greater, men more than women likely to die.
Covid-19 is a deadly virus and among the underprivileged, casualties high.

We started the week at 20,000, now it's 27,000 and rising.
We're going to be worst hit in Europe which somehow isn't surprising.

No checks at the airports, we were slow to react, PPE in short supply,
Tests not available, herd immunity considered. So why do we wonder why?

Indecision, indecisive behaviour, so much fumbling in the dark.
Should masks be worn? No, they shouldn't. Yes, they should. A totally ridiculous lark.

Weather's been mixed this week, showers with bursts of sunshine.
Gardening replaced by jigsaws and manure by a glass of wine.

Week 7
May 8th 2020

It's been 'Test, track and trace' all week, that's the week seven slogan.
Isle of Wight NHSX app trials started, but success is uncertain.

Isn't trace a synonym of track? Shouldn't the word isolate be included?
No, it's much better if it sounds good, truth is far better occluded.

The app gives us hope, it could bring the R rate down,
If contacts are found fast and isolated when found.

It's been a week of records, some we could well do without.
UK deaths second in the world - what's that all about?

Covid-19 is a pernicious disease with so many varied effects.
Asymptomatic in some but can bring organ failure and deaths.

Advice is to take paracetamol, lie prone, take deep breaths, then cough.
Use an oximeter to measure oxygen levels, but is all that enough?

We've discovered men and women of colour are twice as likely to die.
We must quickly work out what's happening, not just sit and wonder why.

We must try to unravel the virus' impact and understand how it works,
Try different treatments, test drugs and discover how to combat its quirks.

SARS-CoV-2 is destructive. It affects the whole body, often creating a chain.
It can affect anything from lungs to the blood, heart, kidneys, guts and the brain.

Anti-inflammatory drugs are now given to help fight a cytokine storm.
Plasma antibodies given to the severely ill, so many new treatments are born.

Interferon Beta is given to activate immune system and help the virus to be suppressed.
DNA and blood groups are being identified. Different susceptibilities we must test.

75 years ago, war with Germany ended with Germany's unconditional surrender.
TV programmes filled our day with memories, memories so sad but so tender.

But celebrations couldn't be as had been arranged for Friday the 8th of May.
There could be no parades or street parties, but when it's VE Day, there's a way.

Winston Churchill's speech was broadcast and our dear Queen addressed the Nation.
'VE Day 75, the People's Celebration', from Buckingham Palace a great presentation.

Two minutes silence at 11 am led by Prince Charles and Camilla too.
Red Arrows left trails across skies of London, National colours red, white and blue.

In Edinburgh, Cardiff and Belfast, Typhoons were a spectacle when they flew over.
And a lone Spitfire was watched by many as it flew over the white cliffs of Dover.

Police have handed out over 9,000 fines to those guilty of lockdown-breaking.
Motorists have been speeding on motorways; there's fun there for the taking.

A driver drove 130mph on the M25 and another 151mph on the straighter M1.
One clocked up a dangerous 70mph in 20-mile restriction with no thought for anyone.

The weather started overcast this week, but we had a bright spell in the middle.
Boris gave us his 'roadmap', plan for reopening society. Let's hope it doesn't lead to a pickle.

The Archers are all repeats. There's nothing exciting our days to brighten.
Although spring is making changes to our gardens as colours start to heighten.

Seedlings are ready to plant out but frosty nights are still a threat.
Can we rely on just a roll of fleece our frost tender plants to protect?

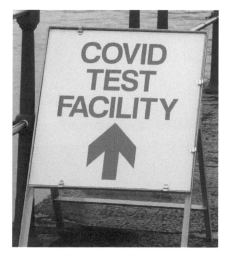

Covid-19 testing centre

The Silence of Lockdown

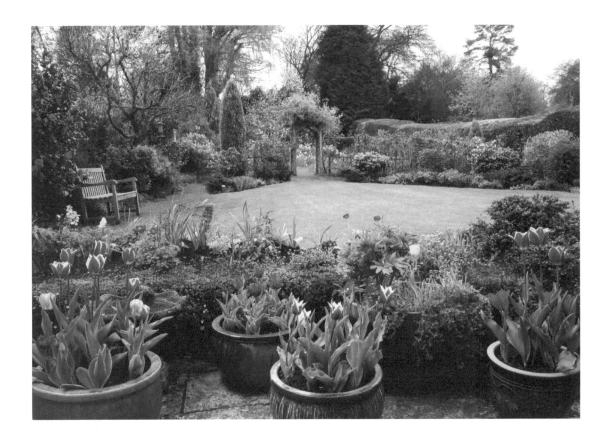

So quiet you can hear a tulip petal fall
A bee buzzes by on its way to somewhere
A faint breeze rustles the leaves in tall trees
A blackbird delights with a medley of songs
A sparrow brightly trills
Silence falls.
The gentle warble of a pigeon breaks the silence
No sound of voices, no dogs barking
Not a plane in the sky or a car passing by
No loud drumming from a car with the window wound down
No lawnmower droning, or water flowing
A rare moment of silence in a fresh and fragrant garden
How can it be so quiet?
You can almost hear the silence.

Week 8
May 16th 2020

A cold wind chilled the country at the beginning of week eight.
Our spirits rose in anticipation with lockdown ease in hot debate.

On Sunday in a short statement, Boris gave us a brand-new slogan.
Our anticipation peaked, but plummeted; we were thrown into confusion.

'Stay Alert, control the virus, save lives', that's how the slogan read.
Slogan 'Stay at home, protect the NHS, save lives' now safely put to bed.

But what is meant by 'Stay Alert'? was the cry across the country.
As advice to cross the road it's fine, to avoid a deadly virus but perfunctory.

On Wednesday, Prime Minister Johnson the meaning of 'Stay Alert' made clear.
'Stay at home, go to work, wash your hands, social distance. No less confusing we fear.

But 'Stay at home' it didn't mean, although that may have been more wise.
It means move house, visit garden centres, drive somewhere and exercise.

Now don't forget to go to work, if you can't do your work at home.
But remember not to take public transport; you must walk, cycle or drive alone.

If you must take public transport then cover your face, don't ask,
Yes, gone is the advice it does no good, don't think about wearing a mask.

We're lucky for we're allowed to meet just one friend in a public park.
Not at home or in our own garden and two metres must we stay apart.

On Thursday there was excitement - an antibody test has been approved.
Swiss pharmaceutical company Roche has done it, all doubt has been removed.

The test is 'highly specific'. Almost 100% accurate even.
At last, we'll now know who's had Covid but lasting immunity's still unproven.

Alarming to hear 100 children have a strange disease to Covid-19 linked.
With fever, rash and inflammation, all symptoms are quite distinct.

Research continues across UK. Covid-19 storm cloud has a silver lining.
Genetic code of patients is analysed. The varied reaction needs defining.

Edinburgh University, Genomics England and NHS together hope to perfect
Analysis of a patient's genome to make infection severity possible to predict.

The week warmed up towards the end, in fact, it became quite hot.
We embraced the sun but frost damage was done. Gardens had suffered a lot.

We're grateful as we can all go out now, but the threat of Covid-19 still remains,
We must just remember to 'stay alert', wash our hands and not take buses or trains.

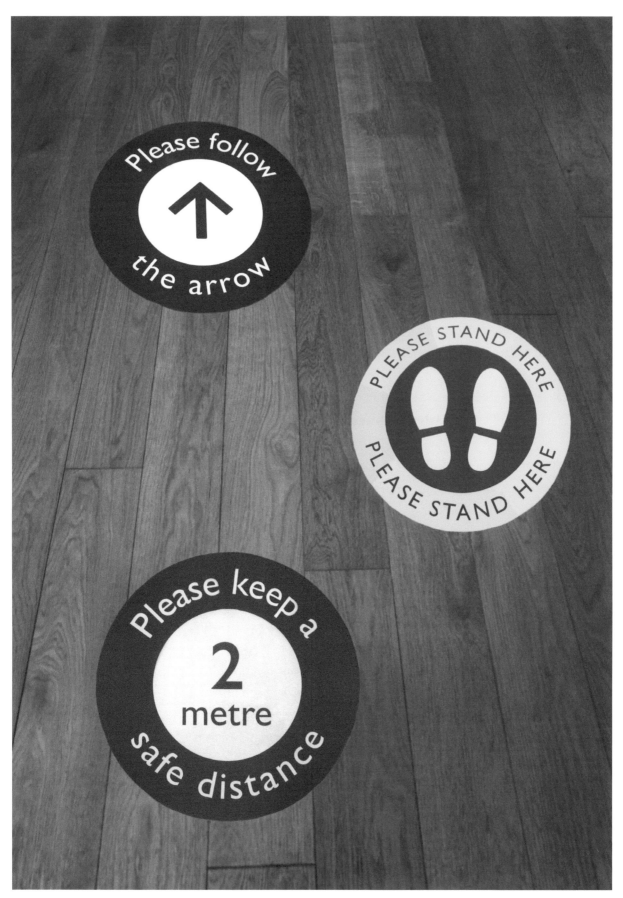

Signs found on floors during pandemic.

Week 9
May 23rd 2020

Week nine sizzled in with record temperatures getting us all steamed up.
Gardens gasped and beaches heaved, social distancing was right out of luck.

Government says schools to reopen June 1st, maybe. It put schools in quite a spot.
Some say 'that's impossible', so should schools go back soon or should they not?

Cambridge is the first university to spell out a roadmap with less fun.
Lectures will be online for all the academic year from 2020 to 2021.

Hydroxychloroquine and chloroquine are in the news once more.
Trump is taking hydroxychloroquine, but as a prophylactic, not a cure.

The world takes on trials for these drugs; can they Covid's inflammation tame?
UK joins in, starts Remdesivir trials too, an anti-viral Gilead drug of fame.

T-cells which fight infection found to be depleted in those severely ill.
Cytokine storms decrease T-cells, for a cure, Roche's Actemra has appeal.

Trial of new swab test for coronavirus in Hampshire's A & E departments has been started.
With results in 20 minutes, it will revolutionize swab tests should results prove to be trusted.

Sad news that nearly one-third of deaths have in care homes now occurred.
Untested residents sent back from hospital; such behaviour quite absurd.

More symptoms of Covid-19 have at last by authorities been accepted,
Loss or change of smell or taste can mean by Covid-19 you've been infected.

Each day we're blinded by statistics, only some of interest, it could be said.
But 5% in UK have had Covid-19 and 17% in London; a much more interesting thread.

Hamster research proves that use of masks could be worth their weight in gold.
Hamsters don't actually wear the masks - a mask partition between cages works we're told.

Airlines are 'up in arms', a fourteen-day quarantine for arrivals is to be brought in.
It's a bit late to introduce it now and death to the travel industry it may well begin.

Captain Tom Moore has popped up once again, now a centenarian of renown.
He'll be knighted in the autumn, wonderful recognition by the crown.

St Paul's Cathedral has started a 'Book of Remembrance' for those who died.
Photos and memories of all loved ones lost will now online be supplied.

As week nine ends, the weather is cooler and strong winds blow in the trees.
Courgettes are setting, broad beans are growing. We can't wait to try the peas.

Week 10
May 30th 2020

Cummings-Gate broke start of week ten. Senior advisor and government rule-maker
Drove 260 miles to Durham, in lockdown, while Covid-infected. Now a rule-breaker.

Cummings had no regrets and Boris supported him, responsibility so carelessly discarded.
The public burned white-hot with anger, feeling their many sacrifices had been disregarded.

On his wife's birthday, to Barnard Castle he drove, his faulty eyesight to put to the test.
From hospital his wife and son he collected, we're not sure we'll ever really know the rest.

Cummings won't resign, Boris won't sack him. Our objections ignored, we're fit to bust.
Boris, now damaged by supporting Cummings, has totally lost all the people's trust.

By Wednesday, Boris did us implore to put Cummings behind us, not at his front door.
But worries arose that things had now changed. People may no longer respect the law.

Primary schools to reopen June 1st, but it will be for nursery, first and sixth years only.
Car showrooms and open markets will join them. Let's hope it's not all very much too early.

Maybe June 15th non-essential shops will reopen but only if they're Covid-19 secure.
It depends on the R number, so we've been told, less than one it must be, not more.

From next Monday, we can have a picnic for six, sitting two metres apart in the garden.
Just don't go inside to use the loo, because if you do, you'll find cleaning is part of the bargain.

Test, trace and isolate on Thursday started, short notice was given so few were ready.
If symptoms develop you must get a test. Your close friends when contacted won't be merry.

If for 15 minutes they've been within 2 metres of you, they must totally isolate for 14 days.
Never mind if they're working and will not get paid, it's their civic duty to comply anyway.

Exciting news - Gilead's Remdesivir has been passed. It can be used by the NHS.
It stops the virus multiplying, shortens recovery time. We hope it's a tremendous success.

WHO trials for hydroxychloroquine have stopped; it was causing heart problems, even deaths.
It treats Malaria well but Covid puts a strain on the heart, which made it unlikely to pass the test.

We went into the week with 36,793 deaths, a number that brings us no credit.
On Friday the figure was up 1,377, let's point the finger of blame, but who will get it?

Cheltenham races, Liverpool's football match too, created hot spots and should've been cancelled.
Skiers flowed back through airports, no instructions to quarantine, negligence truly unparalleled.

Too little PPE, testing unavailable where needed, care homes forced to take positive patients.
The list is endless, lack of planning obvious, such gross incapability to make sensible arrangements.

It's been hot this week, the gardens still gasp, with no rain we've had to water every day.
The water board noticed that demand has gone up and in six months we'll have to shell out and pay.

But we're enjoying the sunshine and life in the garden is simple, do we need to do anything else?
Entertaining is complicated. It may not be worthwhile, so settle down and enjoy peace by yourself.

JUNE 2020

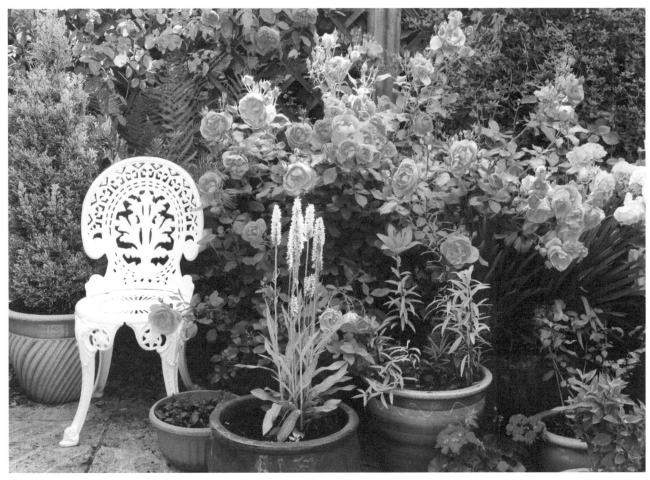

Roses, wild orchids and lilies in summer garden.

Week 11
June 6TH 2020

Is lockdown ease happening too quickly? Start of week 11 raised many people's concern.
Independent SAGE scientists are worried, think government's undue haste they should spurn.

'Test, track and isolate' is in its infancy, app not operational, far more testing is needed yet.
Five tests complete but level three not reached, all conditions have still not even been met.

Some primary schools have restarted, attendance only 40% -70%, quite low.
Temperatures are taken, hands washed on arrival. We must wait to see how things go.

Social distancing with children quite a challenge. Staff praised for how they have coped.
Only fifteen per class, wigwam built as extension, bubble system to keep pupils apart.

Ikea, on its first day of opening, created a new day out for families and friends.
Queue in a car park for three hours in dodgy fresh air. Pleasurable? Well, that all depends.

Monday this week shielded people allowed to go out; they've been granted freedom at last.
They can go out with one person to keep them company with feelings of joy unsurpassed.

By Wednesday, Keir Starmer had had enough. He told PM, 'Stop winging it, get a grip'.
PM denied incompetence, said he'd acted at the right time, infection numbers were starting to dip.

Anti-inflammatory drug Ibuprofen, as lipid capsule, to be tested, trials underway.
The hope is it will reduce respiratory failure, decrease need for ventilation and hospital stay.

Wearing of face covering on public transport will be mandatory June 15th, such a novel idea!
Fines for non-compliance, transport may be denied, so get your sewing kit out, make your own gear.

Hospitals had a big shock when at the end of the week the government did suddenly tell,
All hospital staff must wear masks all the time, all visitors and outpatients as well.

More bonkers ideas from the government - 14 days quarantine for travellers to start on Monday.
Bizarre that 'Arrivals' from low infection countries must quarantine in a growingly infected UK.

On Thursday the streets were quiet; no sound of clapping for the NHS anymore.
It was good to give thanks on a Thursday and meet neighbours outside the front door.

Only one-third of dentists will start work on Monday. Too little notice for preparation was given.
A mere 5 to 10 emergency patients to be seen each day. Normal service resumption still uncertain.

Report by Public Health England said deaths from Covid in ethnic minority groups is high.
Asians, Chinese and Caribbeans affected badly, but Bangladeshis twice as likely to die.

At the end of the week, we're ashamed to report over 40,000 loved ones from Covid-19 have died,
Over 90% of deaths in the over-65 age group. Over 70s take great care should you want to survive.

It's sad the way things are going, dissension and bad news getting harder to take,
On the bright side, there's flour in the shops now, so put your pinnies on, get starting to bake.

It's been cooler this week, in fact quite cold, we've had to put those thick winter woollies back on.
We've had a drop of rain, not enough to fill water butts. Where's all that lovely sunshine gone?

Tomatoes are growing and there are freshly picked courgettes for supper tonight.
But as one in eight households has no outside space, gardening's a privilege, not a right.

So, let's sit down and count our blessings. We've had a beautiful summer so far.
Things are bound to get better soon, then we can eat out and have a drink at the bar.

Week 12
June 13TH 2020

U-turn from the government at start of week 12, now schools won't reopen as planned.
Plans for all ages to start too ambitious. They'll go back in September and not beforehand.

Social distancing in small spaces impossible, there simply isn't enough room.
They'll have to stay at home and study, use the internet or catch up on Zoom.

Some members of parliament say the 2-metre rule should be reduced to one,
To help schools to reopen and businesses restart, say it needs to be swiftly done.

Children can't go to school but on the bright side can enjoy trips to safari parks or zoos.
Parents will welcome release from teacher slavery, now there's something else they can do.

The mood isn't good in England. The government is losing the people's support.
Excuses don't explain poor decisions; defensiveness not an appropriate retort.

Body of over 400 families who've lost loved ones say government must face enquiry.
Too many have died, poor decisions cost lives, the government the blame they should carry.

Half of lost lives could have been saved, say scientists, if lockdown was just one week earlier.
Borders were kept open, no quarantine imposed, nothing short of a catastrophic blunder.

With envy, we regard Guernsey, Isle of Man and New Zealand as they have no cases at all.
Early lockdown, efficient tracking, quarantining, closed borders all created effective firewall.

On Wednesday, Boris led the briefing, told of plans for household bubbling he'd devised.
Those living alone can create bubble with one household; social distancing for them revised.

Lone grandmothers or grandfathers will be happy to hug all their grandchildren once again.
Read them bedtime stories and stay overnight - such joy they'll find hard to contain.

Now singles can at last get together, meet in person, touch each other, not just date online.
The imagination runs wild, so much fun to be had, their happiness will soar to cloud nine.

Churches will open for private prayer only, no services or singing allowed.
Things are getting better, there is no doubt, but is it in a manner for which we are proud?

Test and Trace is up and running, results published for the very first week.
31,000 contacts found from 8,000 tested but one third tested couldn't be reached.

85% of those contacted agreed to self-isolate, but it's not really quite what we'd hoped.
Things should get better as we get used to the system and people learn how to cope.

We've had plenty of rain this week and the gardens at least have been happy.
But we can't sit outside in the rain with four friends, have fun and enjoy being chatty.

So much sunshine in May we all loved and enjoyed, it was certainly a wonderful perk.
Please come back soon or we'll have to stay inside, swap gardening for boring housework.

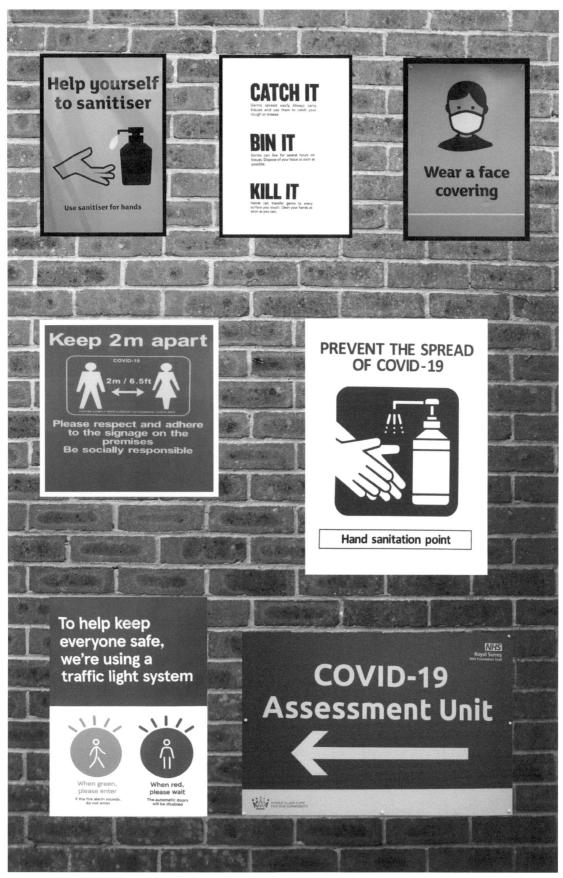

Signs and posters displayed during pandemic

Week 13
June 20ᵗʰ 2020

Non-essential shops open, masks popping up everywhere. Week 13 so full of change.
With a massive U-turn, masks essential in hospitals, on ferries, buses, trains and planes.

EasyJet is back in the air, no cabin service but an individual call for your personal slot in the loo.
Loos spread infection so put down the lid when you flush, in public loos, it's essential to do.

Many sports have resumed but behind closed doors, difficult for pigeon racing it's true.
Royal Ascot with no people, but at home in top hats people chose a virtual version to view.

Oxford vaccine is in its second phase, results in autumn, we hope, if it goes as expected.
AstraZeneca are preparing to make 400,000 doses to save us all from becoming infected.

Imperial College started vaccine trials too, for a vaccine developed a very different way.
Two million doses held in a one-litre bottle can be manufactured worldwide, so they say.

The cheap anti-inflammatory steroid drug Dexamethasone, we're pleased to say, passed its trials.
It will save a fifth of patients on oxygen, a third on ventilation, is administered in pill form or phials.

Scientists, economists, politicians will get together for a two-metre formal review.
Reducing two to one would help schools go back as long as it doesn't increase infections too.

A week of government U-turns, but that's not all bad, meal vouchers for children in need.
NHS tracking app scrapped in favour of the Google-Apple app, let's hope it progresses with speed.

Good news from Matt Hancock - the Covid-19 alert level to be lowered from four to three.
He declared it as a 'big moment for the country'; what difference will it make? Well, we'll see.

We're all keeping busy finding things to do, although the garden has looked after itself in the main.
Nice to entertain family at two-metre distance; an extra big gazebo is needed to hide from the rain.

One furloughed worker had a novel idea, six duck eggs she bought fresh from Waitrose.
Put them in an incubator, three fluffy ducklings hatched, now what on earth will she do with those?

The weather's been changeable all week, we've had thunderstorms and plenty of rain.
The garden is happy but we're rather cold, perhaps it's time to book a quick trip to Spain.

The week's gone okay with a few highs and lows and things are getting better each day.
Let's hope it continues and the rules we're now following will safely keep the coronavirus at bay.

Week 14

June 27th 2020

Wow! Start of week 14 we heard about a new way of living, just in England, from the 4th of July.
From 'Super Saturday' there will be countless things we can do, fun available in endless supply.

A meal out in a Perspex bubble, a gin and tonic or a pint of your favourite brew,
Stay the night, if you like, but if it's a haircut you need, then you won't be the first in the queue.

Why not get married with up to 30 guests, or attend a service in church without any singing?
Libraries await, community centres will open, bingo hall beckons if your buzz is from winning.

Funfairs, adventure parks, amusement arcades and theme parks open for laughter and a bit of fun.
Thinking's your bag? Then galleries, museums and cinemas will help to get plenty of thinking done.

If it's the kids you want to amuse then try child-friendly activities, enjoy a super family day out.
Zoos, safari parks, aquariums, farms or a model village will amuse them, of that there is little doubt.

But disappointment abounds as beauticians, gyms and swimming pools all stay firmly shut.
If it's a tattoo you're after to remember the virus, then you are most definitely clean out of luck.

Do you have a desire to go somewhere? Then pack your suitcase, a UK holiday is waiting for you.
Caravan parks, hotels and guest houses are open. Any with spotlessly clean facilities will do.

If you can't wait until 'Super Saturday', pack, then head to the airport and jump on a plane.
From last Sunday, quarantine was removed and tourists are very welcome in sunny old Spain.

To make this work social distancing has changed, cut from two metres to one metre plus.
But it comes with 'mitigation', the government's word of the week, without it it's far too dangerous.

What's 'mitigation' then we ask? It's the act of making a condition or consequence less severe.
Reducing social distancing to 'one metre plus' comes with risks, so precautions are needed, it's clear.

No face-to-face seating, good ventilation, face coverings and handwashing facilities are a must.
Restaurants play soft music so that no one needs to shout. It will reduce virus transfer we can trust.

Two households can get together indoors but social distancing must be observed all the time.
You'll need to rotate your friends, try them all out indoors and enjoy a social distanced glass of wine.

The heat has been building this week; on Thursday at Heathrow, it reached centigrade 34.4.
Half a million people packed onto the sand in Bournemouth - a major incident declared. That is poor.

We need to balance risk to live with the virus for the foreseeable future, or so we've been told.
Thirteen vaccines worldwide in trial and if one of them works our thanks in spades we'll unfold.

'None of us is safe until all of us are safe'. It was the UN Secretary-General who said that.
One in 1,700 is infected so social distancing and fewer contacts make us safer, an indisputable fact.

Now, ladies, it's time to invest in a larger handbag because there's a lot of gear you have to put in it.
Masks (at least two), alcohol hand wipes (two packs) and bottle of sanitiser are the necessary kit.

Thunderstorms and rain are forecast for this weekend, but then at least we'll escape from the heat.
So, let's sit back, relax, enjoy the last of the sun and if we're peckish rustle up something tasty to eat.

JULY 2020

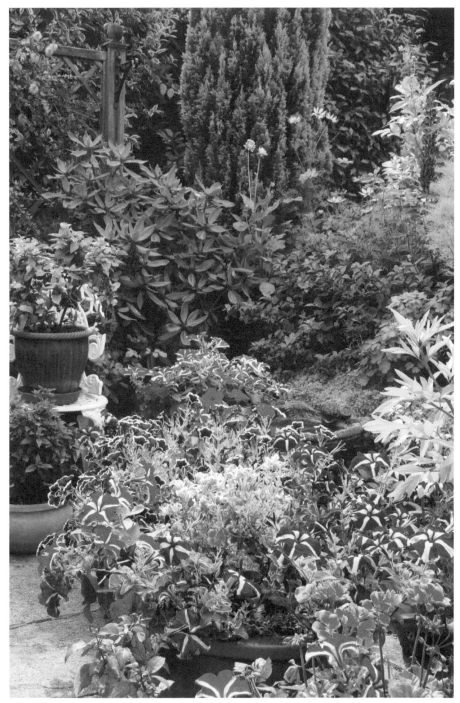

Patio pots full of petunias and geraniums

Week 15
July 4th 2020

Oh dear! It's week 15 and in Leicester, there's a spike of that dreaded virus organism.
An uncompromising SARS–CoV-2 virus has refused to comply with our British optimism.

Super Saturday is here but 'lockdowned' Leicester can't be part of our joyous celebration.
Barnsley, Bradford, and Rochdale are in danger of joining Leicester in their desperate situation.

With pubs opening on a Saturday night, thirst for three months unsatiated and unquenched,
Will alcohol flow too freely and Covid caution with good sense from drinkers be quickly wrenched?

Hairdressers have wasted no time to right those bad coronavirus hair days, our lovely locks return.
Some of them opened at midnight with appointments in the wee small hours of Saturday, we learn.

All schools will return in September; our ministers have hatched a cunning plan with bubbles.
Primary schools, 1 for each class, secondary schools, 1 per year, their numbers more than doubled.

Two Covid cases within 14 days will burst a safety bubble and pupils must return to lonely isolation.
Test kits supplied by schools and mobile units for bad outbreaks form part of this latest innovation.

'Foreign and Commonwealth Office advice against all but essential travel' from 10th July is lifted.
Holidays abroad are possible once more, travellers can return, quarantine rules have shifted.

74 countries can come to the UK but they don't all want us, so plan where you holiday with care.
Make sure when you make that holiday choice that it's to a country that will welcome you there.

The government has struggled over quarantine. Air bridges and travel corridors just disappeared.
Their traffic light system, red for U.S., Russia, China and Portugal evaporated in hours, 'twas weird.

Welsh and Scottish first ministers both declared our government planning lamentable, shambolic.
Decisions are made, they say, but with no planning for implementation. A method like this is chronic.

The world is up in arms. Trump has bought up all 500,000 doses of the Gilead drug Remdesivir.
At £1,900 a course, it's expensive; at least Dexamethasone is £5 a course, cheap, available and here.

Blood plasma with antibodies, a treatment under trial, has good results already from transfusions.
High-level donors, males of Asian background once severely ill, can provide the best donations.

Over 100 vaccines are in development worldwide, seventeen have human trials already underway.
Many countries working hard, development to production 12 -18 months, we hope there's no delay.

It's been windy this week with gale-force winds and blustery showers beating our flowers around.
Gentle rose petals torn and scattered by heartless winds have caused garden damage so profound.

But at least we've had some rain and our gardens are green, flowers happy with a welcome drink.
Life's not so bad, we can start to plan a holiday, go somewhere nice, or at least that's what we think.

Week 16
July 11th 2020

Into the early hours of Sunday, pubs were packed, social distancing dispatched by drunken clusters.
Police reported happy drunks, angry drunks, fights and naked men but also some perfect punters.

Sunday at 5 pm, week 16, we clapped again. 72 years of our beloved NHS to celebrate.
We clapped for carers who put their lives at risk to fight the virus, dedication we couldn't emulate.

On Tuesday three pubs closed. Saturday drinkers with new symptoms told landlords of the fact.
90 customers were contacted by one pub, contact details taken helped them to be very quick to act.

Office of National Statistics found 80% of cases testing positive were actually asymptomatic.
Some later developed symptoms but infection without symptoms is dangerous and problematic.

Regular testing will start in hospitals and care homes soon. Asymptomatic cases will be sought out.
Staff tested once a week, residents each month. 20,000 care home deaths tragic there is no doubt.

'Too many care homes didn't really follow the procedures in the way they could have,' Boris bleated.
Owners exploded; such unjust and outrageous accusations. Their reactions were fiery and heated.

Virus aerosols survive in the air for up to 16 hours we've heard, a perfect way to spread infection.
Masks worn in shops, public transport and badly ventilated rooms are a common-sense protection.

Rishi Sunak gave away £30 billion in his cunning Covid budget and splashed the cash to praises sung.
Businesses to be paid £2,000 for creating apprentice jobs in a 'Kick Start' programme for the young.

£1,000 bonus to employees who take furloughed workers back. It's a welcome drop of nectar.
Stamp duty holiday for houses up to £500,000 should kick start businesses in the housing sector.

VAT only 5% for hospitality and attractions. It will last 6 months, to encourage people back.
In August take the family out, 50% discount, up to £10 a head. Enjoy an 'Eat out to help out' snack.

There will be no pantomimes at Christmas. Indoor theatres won't raise their curtains until 2021.
But from Saturday outdoor theatres and pools open. If the weather's warm that could be fun.

For tattooists, spas, tanning salons and beauticians, (no facials), Monday is their opening date.
Leisure centres, indoor pools, sports halls and gyms will open July 25th, so these will have to wait.

On Thursday, sad news - John Lewis and Boots shops will shut, putting thousands out of work.
Eight John Lewis stores and 48 Boots opticians will close their doors and cause redundancy havoc.

The Covid risk is less they say. Cases are only one per 3,000 of population but it's still not a total fix.
So, take care what you choose to do as there's high risk, low risk but seldom is there ever no risk.

The weather wasn't great this week. With gardens soaked and windswept, no way we could sit out.
Next week the weather should get better, sunshine will make us happy and that's what it's all about.

Week 17
July 18th 2020

Start of week 17, Blackburn with Darwen virus spike identified and lockdown measures selected.
South Asians in terraced housing with high occupancy have led to entire households being infected.

Leicester's restrictions ease from 24th July, schools go back but bars and restaurants won't reopen.
Hot spots identified, lockdown restrictions put in place is the Boris 'whack-a-mole' strategy chosen.

Masks, or should we say face coverings, not really sure, but whatever they are they're mandatory,
In shops from 24th July and on public transport. 'Useless in an office,' confirms the Health Secretary.

Treat them like your socks, we're told. Wash them with your normal wash, once daily, it's essential.
They'll be worn for the foreseeable future, or until we have a vaccine. We hope they're beneficial.

So, ladies, skip the lipstick, there's a saving to be had right there. Load on the eye make-up instead.
For the deaf and hard of hearing relying on lip-reading it's difficult, harder to understand what's said.

To fight an airborne virus, masks make sense. Shouldn't they have been introduced earlier we ask?
Washing hands and singing 'Happy Birthday' not enough to cope with the deadly coronavirus task.

Boris has committed to an independent enquiry into the government's handling of the pandemic.
It's criticised for muddled messaging, poor planning with no clear strategy and efficiency hardly epic.

Renewed hope for Oxford vaccine, immune response in volunteers, T-cells and antibodies produced.
'Cosy Bear', Russian intelligence group, hacking into vaccine research has made for alarming news.

Studies show 1 in 7 severely ill patients develop heart damage. Medical studies go on at pace.
Antibody infusion possible for the vulnerable if no vaccine before winter. It may help us in the race.

Southampton University has a saliva test on trial, tests once a week, processing in just 20 minutes.
Virus shows up in saliva first making early diagnosis possible. A test, we hope, with many benefits.

Boris, in his road map on Friday, announced more power to councils for local lockdown measures.
They have power to close shops, pubs, restaurants, cafés, parks, events and other local pleasures.

'Hope for the best, plan for the worst'. Maybe 'significant return to normality' possibly for Christmas.
'Use public transport', go back to work when employers think its best is the potted PM's message.

But badly ventilated offices aren't Covid-secure, although filters in air conditioning can help a little. Newly developed lights fitted with safe levels of UV that kill the virus will make office safety simple.

On Friday, the Queen knighted Captain Sir Tom Moore at Windsor Castle in a personal ceremony. On the lawn, with her father's sword, she knighted Tom who raised £32.7 million for NHS charities.

The weather's been all up and down this week. Wind, rain, sunshine and chilliness all on the cards. But we could still sit outside and entertain with social distancing in our gardens or backyards.

No longer do we look into an abyss of nothingness; there's plenty for us to do and holidays to plan. But take care, remember Covid safety if you venture out to sea in a boat or on roads in a caravan.

Week 18
July 25th 2020

Oxford vaccine, ChAdOx1 nCov19, has passed its safety trials. Week 18 brings us encouraging news.
Side effects only mild fever and headache, treatable with paracetamol says one of Lancet's reviews.

Oxford vaccine is derived from a chimpanzee common cold virus made safe through modification.
Genetic instructions for Coronavirus 'spike protein', the cell invader, transferred to the vaccination.

Vaccine triggered immune response in 1,077 volunteers. Killer T-cells were produced in 14 days,
Antibodies in 28. For proof that it provides protection, we must wait until the end of the third phase.

2,000 volunteers in S. Africa, 5,000 in Brazil, 10,000 in UK, 30,000 in USA will take part in phase 3.
Two doses give stronger immune response but for how much immunity is needed we'll wait to see.

Production of vaccine by AstraZeneca has already started in the hopes it can the coronavirus repress.
UK has ordered 100 million doses; they'll have to pay even if the vaccine isn't a complete success.

The Government have also ordered 30 million of the German vaccine and 60 million of the French;
As 9 in 10 vaccines usually fail, it's an insurance policy, help our urgent thirst for a vaccine to quench.

The PM has just announced that 50% of the population before winter will be given free flu vaccine.
It will stop confusion with the covid virus but how many people take up the offer remains to be seen.

On Friday, masks, or face coverings became mandatory in shops, banks and take-away food outlets.
Staff, disabled and children under 11 are all exempt. For non-compliance, a fine of £100 you'll get.

Waitrose check customers before they enter, Tesco are selling masks at the entrance to the store.
Sainsbury's will turn a blind eye, say nothing, but other shops will hand out free masks at the door.

Only one in 7 people are against mask-wearing and we hope it will give us more confidence to shop.
Hard if you're a chocolatier relying on the delicious smell to sell and a sample in each mouth to pop.

If you wear a turban or have a long beard, putting it on successfully will take some perseverance.
Trump, with a sudden change of heart, urges Americans to wear masks if unable to social distance.

Boris said 'there were things we could have done differently'. There were 'lessons to be learned'.
He told Laura Kuenssberg no one understood coronavirus when he was interviewed and questioned.

Southampton research with Synairgen carried out Interferon beta trials hoping Covid-19 to suppress.
If delivered by nebuliser as a fine mist then 79% of patients were less likely to develop severe illness.

The weather's been pleasant this week but perhaps we didn't have quite enough rain for the garden.
Water butts are emptying but vegetables flourishing and the flowers creating a colourful haven.

Outside entertaining as evenings grow cooler find shivering guests, once chilled, lose their spark.
A patio heater is perfect for sitting outside eating and makes supping wine possible until dark.

AUGUST 2020

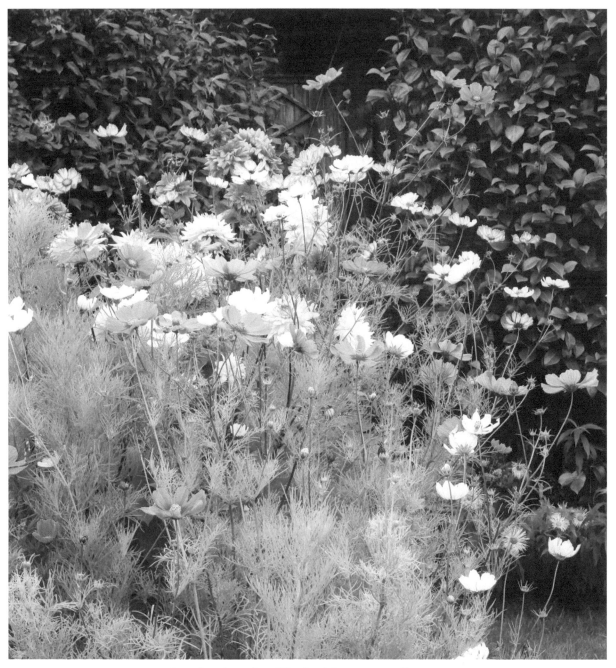

Garden border filled with cosmos flowers.

Week 19
August 1ˢᵗ 2020

Week 19 and we've been told to exercise more, get on our bikes to solve the UK obese crisis.
A £50 voucher for 50,000 bikers is on offer to fix broken bikes. It's on a first-come, first-serve basis.

Two-thirds of us are overweight; junk and unhealthy food blamed for UK's weight increase.
Research shows we're 40% more likely to die or be severely ill with Covid if overweight or obese.

Holiday-makers from Spain, Balearics and Canary Islands must quarantine on return for 14 days.
Spike in Spain has upset want-to-be sunbathers who've had to cancel holidays and shorten stays.

Luxembourg quarantine exemption was removed too and other EU countries are now threatened.
Possible second wave in EU puts UK staycations on the cards, should help holiday uncertainly to end.

R number now 0.8 to 1 and rising. 2,800 new cases of Covid each day last week, rising to 4,200 this.
Boris squeezes the brake pedal; hits pause button on lockdown ease. Covid-19 becomes his nemesis.

30 guests at weddings cancelled, beautician's facials too, empty stalls at Goodwood races an anxiety.
Chris Whitty, Chief Medical Officer, says we're near the limit of what can be done to open up society.

Two households in Greater Manchester, W. Yorkshire and Lancashire can't meet indoors or outside.
A spike in the community has led to new measures, sadly just before the Muslim celebration of Eid.

Mosques open but masks must be worn in cinemas, museums, galleries and all places of worship.
Weddings have few guests and a masked bride means they'll be no kiss for the groom on her lips.

New rules if you're suffering from Covid symptoms, you must isolate for 10 days rather than seven.
Boris has a new slogan - 'hands, face, space, get a test', to protect us from the spread of infection.

The poor nation is feeling a bit battered, but then it does have the highest excess deaths in Europe.
Reckless release of patients from hospital to care homes untested just part of this terrible mess up.

More vaccines on order, 60 million doses from GlaxoSmithKline and Sanofi, ready first half of 2021.
They're scaling up manufacture to a billion doses a year. Just one effective vaccine and we've won.

Cardiff research is cracking the virus' genetic code as it changes, using samples from 6,000 in Wales.
D and G variants found, changes could make virus more or less virulent; such very important details.

Siamese cat tested positive after shortness of breath; caught virus from family so don't kiss your cat.
No evidence you can catch Covid-19 from a pet but with a new virus, it's hard to be surer than that.

On Friday, we had 37.8C at Heathrow, hottest day this year and third-warmest day in UK on record.
Thousands of sun-seekers went to Bournemouth, Brighton and Poole. Such crowds we can ill afford.

Why not avoid beaches altogether? Jump off a boat for a swim, should boating be part of your luck.
Or you could stay at home, sun yourself in the garden and water your plants as they start to dry up.

Week 20

August 8th 2020

Week 20, 'Eat out to help out' has started, just as we're dieting, attempting excess weight to lose.
It's a contrary message. One saves livelihoods and the other saves lives, it's up to us to choose.

Government announces a 90-minute swab test for rapid Covid-19 testing, calling it a 'game-changer.'
A cartridge swab kit can be processed in prisons, schools, care homes or surgeries with no danger.

It identifies the RNA, genome code, if present, allowing rapid segregation of anyone infected.
It will start next week. By end of year, production of a million swab kits each month is expected.

Lockdown restrictions were imposed in the City of Aberdeen after cases of Covid-19 rose to 54.
Bars, cafés, restaurants forced to close, visitors forbidden, travel limited for a week, or maybe more.

Home Affairs Select Committee says having no travel quarantine 13th March was a serious mistake.
Travellers returning from hotspots in Italy and Spain escalated infection and worsened outbreak.

The government denies the error, says it was 'led by the science'. But what is the science based on?
With a new virus, no one knows how it will behave. Wouldn't common sense be better relied upon?

There's talk that pubs will have to close when schools start to reopen on a one in, one out basis.
Teenagers can transmit like adults and Test and Trace isn't good enough to prevent further cases.

Lockdown measures reintroduced in Preston from midnight Friday after rise in Covid-19 infections.
Two households can't meet in homes, private gardens, restaurants or cafés to reduce transmission.

Hospital admissions fall as Covid-19 cases rise suggesting younger people are becoming infected.
Lockdown ease July 4th and more contact allowed has led to community transmission, it's suspected.

Travellers from Belgium, Bahamas and Andorra must quarantine for 14 days from 4 am on Saturday.
France's rising infection is being monitored; quarantine a possibility government officials now say.

October's London Marathon, moved from April, will be an elite-only race, thousands disappointed.
2020 Olympics in Japan was delayed until 2021, but a further delay could well be anticipated.

Oxytocin, 'love hormone', is produced when we touch and hug. Social distancing stopped all that.
Advice is to take a warm bath, feel the breeze on your face, soak up sunshine or get a dog or a cat.

For households, there are hugs aplenty, but when living alone there are no hugs day or night.
So, spare a thought for those alone, pick up the phone, FaceTime, or have a go at using Skype.

The weather's been hot and dry this week; we can sit outside under a sunshade, play a game.
It's too hot for gardening and we have to keep watering the plants but we really shouldn't complain.

Week 21

August 15ᵗʰ 2020

Week 21, 'A' level exam results moderated by Ofqual using algorithms is deemed by many a fiasco.
Virus prevented exams being taken. Grades' estimate by teachers down-graded and now far too low.

Students are deprived of university of choice, but mock results will be considered if schools appeal.
Scottish students complained about low grades so teachers' estimates were accepted, a better deal.

Preston enters lockdown measures; separate households can't meet in homes or private gardens.
Under 30s not social distancing is blamed. 'Don't Kill Granny' local authority says, a sobering lesson.

Northampton sandwich factory that makes M & S sandwiches has 300 positive cases of Covid-19.
Northampton could be facing lockdown measures. It's a second week of lockdown for Aberdeen.

On the bright side, enjoy live performances, soft play, go skating, bowling, or at a casino make a pile.
Wedding receptions of 30 guests can sit for a meal indoors. At last, you can get married in style.

Long-awaited facials and eyebrow threading is now allowed, beauticians with businesses are thrilled
But beauticians and hairdressers must wear FFP 2 masks with visors if regulations are to be fulfilled.

Vaccines bought by UK total 340 million shots and deals signed for 90 million further vaccine doses
From Belgium pharmaceutical Janssen and US biotech company Novavax to increase our chances.

Calculation of Covid deaths is revised. Only deaths less than 28 days after positive test are counted.
This conveniently reduces deaths from 46,000 to 41,000 but still far too high leaving many disgusted.

Exodus from France. Thousands of tourists rush to get home before quarantine starts 4 am Saturday.
Quarantine announced for France, Netherlands, Malta, Aruba, Turks and Caicos. A bit late in the day.

Increase in cases testing positive in July is levelling off, even though far more testing is being done.
Surge in September is expected when children return to school and winter rise may be yet to come.

Fewer are being hospitalized or put on ventilation, suggesting a younger group is being infected.
Once severe illness in over-75 age group, now infections less severe as 15 to 44 age group affected.

From an antibody trial, it is estimated that 3½ million people in the UK have already had the virus.
In finger-prick tests sent out to 100,000 volunteers, 6% had antibodies, but results could be bogus.

The weather was dramatic this week with flooding, thunderstorms, heavy showers and fierce heat. Today, gloomy fog has descended with drizzle and it's chilly. Wouldn't 23C and blue skies be a treat?

But with secure holidays at home, a staycation the sensible option, life is good and the sea is warm. In the garden, there are butterflies and honey bees; who cares if there is the odd thunderstorm?

Week 22
August 22nd 2020

Week 22 made 2020 the most disrupted exam year in history with exam results by students rejected.
Attempt to standardize results using algorithm was abandoned and teachers' assessments accepted.

Government shouldn't have to rely on shocked eighteen-year-olds to point out badly flawed system.
Gavin Williamson and Ofqual apologised but algorithms reflecting bias of creators caused scepticism.

15,000 students now have necessary grades for Uni offer and students can choose first choices.
Cap removed on university places, including important medicine, veterinary and dentistry courses.

GCSE results using assessments has led to the number of top grades and passes rising dramatically.
Sixth forms and colleges must find room for increased number but with Covid-19 reduced capacity.

BTEC results have been delayed until next week. Pearson will review grades before proceeding.
2,000 vocational courses are offered for subjects from aeronautical engineering to hairdressing.

Public Health England and NHS Test and Trace combined creating National Institute for Health, NIHP.
Ministers accused of making PHE scapegoat for failings. NIHP to protect us from pandemics, maybe.

Biotech company in conjunction with Cardiff University awarded funding to develop immunity test.
Looking for T-cells that can produce immunity when antibodies no longer detectable is their quest.

Government says it is going to ramp up testing using tests that can be processed within minutes.
Rolled out in autumn, we hope mass testing of population without symptoms will bring us benefits.

Another week of lockdown measures for Aberdeen. Birmingham cases rise, lockdown may happen.
Leicester has some lockdown measures lifted; nail bars, beauty salons and tattoo parlours can open.

In Oldham, Blackburn and Pendle, Covid-19 cases rise, separate households banned from meeting.
Coupar Angus food processing plant has 68 cases. Premises closed, staff and families now isolating.

More countries fall off the travel corridor list - Croatia, Austria, Tobago and Trinidad are all affected.
17,000 holidaymakers in Croatia rush to board planes before Saturday 4 am; they'll return dejected.

But Portugal is back on the corridor list, no need for returning holidaymakers to quarantine now.
But R number has risen in UK, 0.9 to 1.1 today. A bumpy autumn and winter expected somehow.

We haven't heard from Boris lately. He's our Prime Minister and leadership from him we'd welcome.
He's enjoying a staycation in remote Scottish cottage on the coast. Internet is possibly the problem.

Storm Ellen blew us away at the end of the week. Gale force winds sent frail flower petals flying.
Spring high tides caused coastal flooding. Death Valley 54.4C, world record, brought danger of frying.

But we're okay indoors and there's plenty to do. Eating and poetry writing will fill up some time.
There's not so much news this week but enough for a poem, the only problem is making it rhyme.

Week 23
August 29ᵗʰ 2020

Week 22 Government conveyor belt of U turns rolls on. Masks for some schools, it changes rules.
They're made mandatory in corridors and communal places, in hot spots and lockdown area schools.

In Scotland and Wales, masks are mandatory in all secondary schools in indoor communal places.
Headteachers in England will have discretion over use of face coverings to reduce Covid-19 cases.

Test and Trace is taking longer to process results, fails to reach 80% target for tenth week in a row.
Only 72% of positive cases contacted and only 75% of contacts traced. Inadequate and far too slow.

Schools soon to return in England and Test and Trace must be up to speed to track new clusters.
Dundee school closed. Two children got Covid-19 and there were 21 cases amongst the teachers.

Heads roll over exam fiasco. Top civil servant, Jonathan Slatter sacked by Boris, made a scapegoat.
Ofqual boss Sally Collier resigns. Boris Johnson blames a 'mutant algorithm', and that's a quote.

Storm Francis sweeps in, brings heavy rain and winds up to 70mph causing flooding and damage.
But in the US, Hurricane Laura brings 150mph winds, causes destruction that is far more savage.

Gatwick is to cut 600 jobs, almost a quarter of its workforce. It already has one runway closed.
Rolls Royce cuts 9,000 staff worldwide. Mini factory cuts staff through lack of demand it disclosed.

Restrictions eased in parts of northwest England allowing people to mix in different households.
In Aberdeen, households, restaurants and travel restrictions ease. In Leicester, all restrictions hold.

Last night of Proms will play Rule Britannia and Land of Hope and Glory instrumentally, no singing.
Controversy over no words, with 5,272 empty seats in the Royal Albert Hall no singing's more fitting.

Outbreak in Plymouth after group of 30 teenagers return from holiday on island of Zante in Greece.
Celebrated in town, then 11 of them tested positive. Their mild symptoms helped spread disease.

In Hong Kong, second infection in a 33-year-old man recorded. There was an interval of 4½ months.
Second infection different strain and asymptomatic but alarming. We could all get it more than once.

Countries are struck off the safe travel list. It's Switzerland, Jamaica and Czech Republic this week.
Cuba declared safe for travel which is odd as Havana has curfew as new cases of Covid-19 peak.

Red tape to be cut to register vaccine if it works. Health workers trained in readiness so no regrets.
Health professionals to vaccinate include pharmacists, physiotherapists, dentists, midwives and vets.

Cunard's cruises are suspended until March but if you fancy a cruise, it's not as bad as it sounds.
Take a mini-cruise to see up to 5 liners anchored off Bournemouth, from Poole Quay costs only £15.

Has the summer ended? It's getting colder, days are getting shorter and hours of sunshine are less.
But if summer returns, get the latest fashion accessory - smart matching mask to go with your dress.

SEPTEMBER 2020

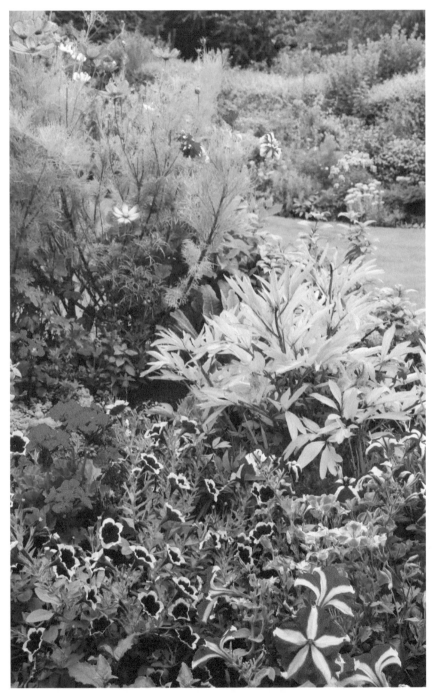

Petunias, geraniums and cosmos in flower

Week 24
September 5th 2020

Week 24. For many, it is back to school full time this week after many months of home-schooling.
Masks worn on school buses, hand sanitiser in bags, together with friends again for some fooling.

Schools look different now, Covid secure with desks in rows and arrows to mark which way to go,
Hand sanitiser everywhere, a work pack on each desk, staggered break times to keep infections low.

New lockdown measures in Greater Glasgow for 800,000, they can't meet in other people's houses.
Infections in UK mostly amongst 18 to 34 age group but admission to hospital lower, say sources.

In north-east, cases rise but Public Health Director says tests have 'dried up, completely evaporated',
Gone to high-risk areas, so low risk depleted, travel 100 miles for test, the distances have escalated.

Londoners sent to Cardiff, Devonians to Carmarthenshire, distance for tests quoted as the crow flies.
Ilfracombe Covid sufferer sent to Swansea. If symptoms include walking on water, it's just 32 miles.

Raves and illegal gatherings arranged all over the country, 500 at rave in Norfolk, 3,000 in Wales.
Organizers fined £10,000 each for arranging them. Equipment confiscated; at least justice prevails.

500 million pounds of government funding to trial saliva test is unveiled. Test takes only 20 minutes.
Southampton Uni and Hampshire schools do trials. Hope to break infection chains with at-home kits.

Scientists developing Oxford vaccine say will know if successful in 6 weeks, they're wonderful geeks.
Biomedica's agreement with AstraZeneca is for 100s of thousands of vaccine doses every 3 weeks.

Planes from Greek islands of Crete and Zante are bringing tons of teenagers home who test positive.
Masks not worn on planes, hundreds have to quarantine, one passenger has dubbed them Covidiots.

Scotland puts Greece and Portugal on quarantine list, Wales names six Greek islands in addition.
England makes no changes to quarantine list at all, making no effort to stop the spread of infection.

'Eat out to help out' serves more than a million meals, restaurants claim 522 million pounds back.
84,700 restaurants signed up for scheme. It helped hospitality; better than giving workers the sack.

Rule Britannia and Land of Hope and Glory will be sung with lyrics on very last night of the proms.
Select group of BBC Singers will sing them; audience asked to take part, to sing along in their homes.

London's Winter Wonderland in Hyde Park has been cancelled, it's sad, it's been going since 2007.
Ice rinks, roller coaster, shows are the fun part, social distancing would remove Christmas heaven.

Soaps are using spouses and partners as body doubles for kissing scenes, they're just using their lips.
That's not as annoying as the Archers' monologues, they're boring and have made interest eclipse.

The garden is less bright now, but dahlias still bloom. It's September, butterflies less likely to flutter.
As weeks pass by, the possibility of an effective vaccine gets closer and that is what really matters.

Week 25
September 12th 2020

Universities return, children start school, workers can go back to work, yet everything isn't okay.
Number of Covid-19 cases dramatically increasing all over the country, over 3,000 new cases a day.

Boris introduces his 'Rule of Six' on Monday. Only six people are allowed to meet indoors and out.
'Rule of Six' applies in Scotland and Wales, with a few differences. £100 fine gives rule more clout.

Marshals will be watching for 'Rule of Six' being broken, they're volunteers and members of council.
They have no powers but can give out masks and hand wipes; must call police if there's any trouble.

The good news is there were 20,000 Covid cases in hospital at the peak but only 837 in hospital now.
Infection mostly in 17–29 age group at present, but it will spread to the vulnerable should we allow.

Universities introduce testing. Cambridge offers students, even without symptoms, tests each week.
Exeter has contract with Halo, first commercial test provider. A saliva test is simple, difficult to beat.

Households can't meet indoors or out in Birmingham, Sandwell and Solihull as now new measures.
R number is above one and cases doubling each week. We could soon be looking at very big figures.

We could take lessons from Belgium. With mini lockdown, they successfully curbed second wave.
Curfew, small gatherings, shop alone, contacts traced and all with cooperation people willingly gave.

Government's 'Moonshot Operation' is born. It's a saliva test for all, results in as little as 20 minutes.
Trials start in Salford in October. Tests each day so people, if negative, may return to normal habits.

That's all well and good but things need improvement right now. Test and Trace isn't working well.
Appointments for drive-through and postal tests aren't available and speed of tests needs to excel.

Oxford vaccine temporarily paused worldwide as volunteer with adverse reaction was hospitalized.
Independent regulator, MHRA, reviews side effects, patient improves but we were so demoralized.

Scotland launched its contact tracing app on Thursday. It's already been downloaded 600,000 times.
England and Wales will launch theirs on September 24th. We need it quickly as the R number climbs.

Government has a new slogan 'Hands, Face, Space'. Why is it we find these slogans so annoying?
We know we need to wash hands, cover face and social distance. It's a habit we're now deploying.

Seven Greek islands removed from safe travel list early this week. Travellers this must not be missed.
Mainland Portugal, Hungary and Réunion removed later. Sweden has now been put back on the list.

Southampton County Council cancelled The International Boat Show only hours before due to open.
230 boats moored on waterfront, 20,000 expected to attend over 10 days. Financial ruin is certain.

No big family gatherings this Christmas. For some households, this may generate a little sigh of relief.
Turkey farmers are worried, no demand for large turkeys; families only needing a small joint of beef.

It felt cooler this week but summer's not yet over, there's a heatwave forecast for next week.
We can warm up again, sit outside in the sunshine and dream up our own government critique.

Week 26
September 19th 2020

Week 26. 'Test and Trace' becomes 'Trace a Test'. Under heavy demand, the system has buckled.
Long queues, no appointments available, no one there to give a test, even when test is scheduled.

Boris promises 500,000 tests by end of October, Matt Hancock promises them in a couple of weeks.
Tests to be prioritised, given first to NHS, care home staff and residents. The system certainly creaks.

Across UK, 13.5 million people are living with restrictions. Belfast and Glasgow now badly affected.
2 million people in north-east in new lockdown measures. In Sunderland, 103 in 100,000 infected.

North West, W. Yorkshire, Midlands and Rhondda Cynon Taf the latest to be put in new measures.
Socializing banned in houses, curfew for pubs and restaurants. It brings many people displeasure.

Over 6,000 Covid cases daily in UK, doubling about every 8 days. Our future's exceedingly worrying.
More people hospitalised, deaths increase to over 20 a day, second wave almost certainly is coming.

30 schools have closed. 300 children sent home to quarantine, from classes and year group bubbles.
There's north-south divide in infection density. London's bad but North has much greater troubles.

Situation in UK is now critical. Boris is considering a 'circuit break' involving hospitality countrywide.
Virus sweeps across Europe. Over 30 million cases worldwide, almost one million already have died.

Test and Trace in England is collapsing, only 50% of all contacts being traced in Manchester to date.
More than a million have downloaded Scotland's new tracing app, 100 people advised to self-isolate.

London's New Year's Eve fireworks are cancelled. Over 100,000 are usually there to enjoy the scene.
Slovenia and Guadeloupe fall off safe travel list, Singapore and Thailand are free from quarantine.

Sarah Gilbert on Radio 4 said if all goes well the vaccine could be ready end of year or start of next.
Oxford restarted its trials after a pause of nearly a week. Our anticipation with anxiety is mixed.

AstraZeneca is able to produce 2 billion doses. Vaccine can be manufactured on a very large scale.
Immune response is produced when antibodies stick to virus spikes and prevent virus entering cells.

New test can diagnose infection in 90 minutes. Developed by DnaNudge, called 'lab-on-a-chip'.
It's used in 8 hospitals. Swab is put in cartridge in shoebox-sized machine, analysed, and that is it.

Italian airport trial started for Covid-free flights on Alitalia from Rome to Milan. We're impressed.
Nasal swab test for passengers, processed in 30 minutes, or you produce evidence of 72-hour test.

Monoclonal antibodies, processed by US company, Regeneron, are being trialled on 2,000 patients.
Antibodies sieved, those that cling best to virus saved, reproduced in lab for effective treatments.

Increasing number of parrots come up for adoption. One owner said, 'they're problematic on Zoom.
They don't repeat things but they're noisy and for business, you really don't need one in the room.'

It's been amazingly hot this week and we should be happy, but the serious situation is concerning.
Hopefully vaccines will come soon then our worries will stop, our future become more appealing.

Week 27
September 26ᵗʰ 2020

Week 27. Bit of a bleak week. Chief Medical Officer and Scientific Advisor gave a gloomy TV briefing.
Estimate is 50,000 Covid cases a day by mid-October, 200 deaths by mid-November. Far-reaching.

New measures from PM. Pubs, bars and restaurants must close at 10pm and offer table service only.
For shop workers, bar staff, waiters and non-seated customers, masks have become mandatory.

Masks are compulsory on public transport. £200 fine for breaking mask-wearing rule when it's law.
Fine for failing to self-isolate after positive test £ 1,000 but, if you do it more than once, a lot more.

Limit on guests at wedding reduced to 15. People asked to work from home. At least it saves on fuel.
UK at tipping point says Matt Hancock. Lockdown can't be ruled out if people don't follow the rules.

UK needs to get R number below 1. It's now between 1.2 and 1.5. Alert level has risen from 3 to 4.
The autumn budget has been cancelled. Very difficult to make decisions while Covid-19 cases soar.

Rishi Sunak announced 'Job Support Scheme'. Starts 1ˢᵗ November when 'Furlough Scheme' spent.
Work 33% minimum in viable job, government tops up wages 22%, salary guaranteed will be 77%.

Jobs must have a future in the short term. Rishi says he can't save every job as finances don't allow.
Night club workers, actors and musicians are among those who must find another job somehow.

Major outbreak in Glasgow Uni, 124 Covid cases and 600 self-isolating. They must by the rules abide.
Scottish students may not go home for Christmas as unlawful for different households to mix inside.

127 cases of Covid at Manchester Metropolitan University, 1,700 students must isolate, stay indoors.
12 UK universities have testing facilities. Nottingham has developed its own and gets our applause.

Test and Trace app launched on Wednesday. More than a million downloaded it first day released.
Detects close contact with Covid case, tells you to self-isolate for 14 days, but voluntary, not policed.

Local restrictions in Swansea, Cardiff and Llanelli. Poor social distancing in 17-24 age group blamed.
11 pm closure for bars and restaurants, can't travel beyond area, households mixing indoors banned.

Novavax vaccine enters phase 3 of trials, produces T-cells and robust antibodies. Enrols 10,000 in UK.
40 promising vaccines being tested globally and 140 in early stages, as officials at WHO happily say.

Oxford scientists develop rapid test using simple colour change, pink to yellow if positive in a blink.
Three vials for each test with different primers, positive test turns two vials yellow, leaves one pink.

UK vaccine human challenge seeks volunteers for January start. They're vaccinated, then infected.
No cure so trial risky, although Remdesivir may help. If successful, shorter route to vaccine expected.

Denmark, Slovakia, Iceland and Curacao are added to travel quarantine list and all airport controls.
Tesco and Morrisons are restricting some items bought. Limit on wet wipes, pasta and toilet rolls.

It became officially autumn this week. It turned windy and chilly so we no longer want to sit outside.
But in Norway, there **is** no bad weather, only bad clothing. So, wrap up and take cold in your stride.

OCTOBER 2020

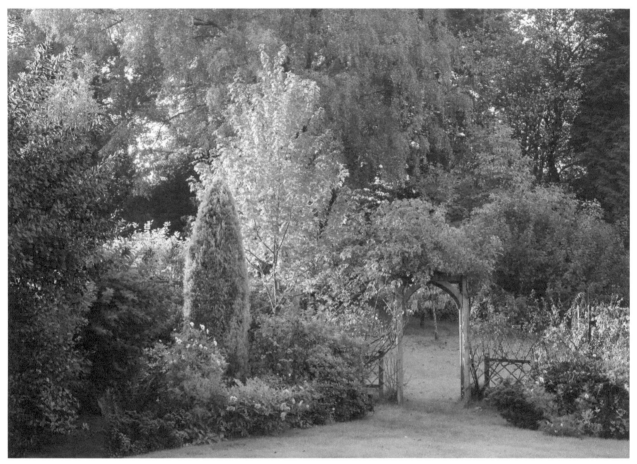

Maple tree glowed with leaves in glorious autumn colours.

Week 29
October 3rd 2020

UK has reached a perilous point. 1 in 4 people is living under restrictions, ¼ of population affected. New measures for Liverpool, Warrington, Middlesbrough and Hartlepool. 268 per 100,000 infected.

Pattern of infection different from first wave. Intensity in second wave concentrated in hotspots. N. East, N. West, Yorkshire and W. Midlands have high infection rates and South Wales also has lots.

Deaths worldwide have reached one million. Nearly half in USA, Brazil and India but UK comes fifth. 80 cases of Covid contracted in Royal Glamorgan Hospital, 8 deaths. Hospital was closed forthwith.

REACT study, Imperial College and Ipsos MORI estimate 1 in 200 with Covid, but spread decreasing. 150,000 randomly selected people tested each month. R number fallen from 1.7 to 1.1, so pleasing.

University of Northumbria confirms 770 students tested Covid positive, only 78 were symptomatic. Students provided with food, laundry and welfare support. Fines for breaking rules were automatic.

Coventry University had hall party with 200 attending. 56 UK universities have cases of coronavirus. Unis will stop face-to-face teaching early, then, after isolating, students can go home for Christmas.

Over 14 million have downloaded the NHS Covid-19 app. Self-isolation if alerted is voluntary. Test and Trace alert to self-isolate has a £1,000 fine, £10,000 maximum, and isolation is compulsory.

Testing of 500 in pork meat processing plant in Cornwall uncovered 170 cases, many asymptomatic. 'Proactive testing' stopped wider spread to community. Much better if testing was more systematic.

Arrivals from Poland and Turkey now have to quarantine. Italy's control of Covid-19 best in Europe. Strict rules, police checks on mask-wearing and fines, plus measures have stopped the virus's gallop.

President Trump and his wife tested positive for Covid-19, started self-isolating in the White House. We wish them well, but aversion to masks and cavalier approach didn't help Trump or his spouse.

24 hours after diagnosis, Trump is transferred by helicopter, Marine One, to Walter Reed Hospital. He's been treated with antiviral drug Remdesivir and Regeneron's experimental antibody cocktail.

'Reckless' SNP member of parliament went by train from London to Glasgow after testing positive. PM's father was seen with no mask in shop. Corbyn attended dinner party for 9. All were defensive.

Government to offer free college courses for all ages, courses for butchers to windfarm technicians.
They'll be of 'A' level standard but won't start until April so there's no need to make hasty decisions.

In Finland, you may be met by a dog at the airport. They're used for sniffing out Covid-19 accurately.
Can pick it up even if symptoms haven't developed and test is negative. That is an amazing capacity.

Stockpilers go from loo rolls to Christmas puddings. Crackers, that's what they'll next be hoarding.
Father Christmas is writing the letters this year. He's writing to Rishi Sunak for help with his funding.

It gets dark earlier now. Weather is wet, cold and windy. Already our gas central heating is humming.
Logs have arrived, Scrabble dusted off and woollies unpacked. We're ready for whatever is coming.

Week 30
October 10th 2020

'It will be bumpy up until Christmas and beyond' says Boris. 38% of ICU beds now have Covid cases.
478 people admitted to hospital in one day, rise of 25%. Two-thirds of cases are in Northern places.

R number between 1.2 and 1.5. It's thought 170 to 240 people in 100,000 have Covid in community.
Hospital admissions are rising. 250,000 cases in UK provide us with evidence of infection's intensity.

Nottingham has 689 virus cases in 100,000, highest in UK. Restrictions will be announced Monday.
Start of tier two restrictions on Wednesday was leaked. Weekend offers the 'last chance to party'.

Pubs and restaurants close across central Scotland for 16 days. It includes Edinburgh and Glasgow.
In rest of Scotland, alcohol is allowed till 10 pm but drinking and drink with dining must be al fresco.

Three-tier system is being considered for England. Tier one existing measures includes 'rule of six'.
In tier three, pubs, restaurants and cafés may close. In tier two, households may not be able to mix.

Rishi announced 'local furlough' scheme to support businesses forced to close due to restrictions.
Two-thirds of salary to be paid as 'safety net'. It will give six months of job support and protection.

Technical glitch for 7 days led to 16,000 positive cases not being reported, or their contacts traced.
The 7,000 cases reported in one day should have been 11,000. Any confidence in system misplaced.

Tens of thousands now suffering from 'long Covid', even after mild illness. Clinics are being set up.
Characterised by crippling fatigue, joint pain, breathlessness and anxiety. Needs to be followed up.

Trump said, 'Don't be afraid of the virus', 'Don't let it dominate your life'. In hospital for only 4 days.
He praised his treatment, wants the same treatment free for everyone. Hopes has he surely raised.

He believes Regeneron's monoclonal antibody cocktail saved him and 'seniors should get it quick'.
Will make sure Eli Lilly's drug license is fast-tracked. He said, 'A blessing from God that I caught it'.

Queen praises media for helpful reporting of virus. Media has provided 'trusted and reliable' news.
It's been a 'vital service' during pandemic and helped old people. News can so easily be confused.

Queen's birthday honours published. 400 workers honoured for their contribution during pandemic.
They were delayed so outstanding people could be recognized - volunteers, key workers and medics.

Paris bars and restaurants close for 2 weeks. Infections above 250 in 100,000 triggered highest alert.
France to extend restrictions to four more cities, Lyon, Lille, Grenoble and Saint-Etienne, for a start.

Bangor has restrictions imposed on entering and leaving city. Households cannot meet indoors.
Good news that five Greek islands have been added to safe travel list. A fine holiday could be yours.

Scientist said surfaces aren't the main cause of virus spreading. Aerosols are cause of the spread.
Masks are important but no need to heat daily newspaper in AGA. It's better used for making bread.

Leaves are falling off the trees and crunching beneath our feet as autumn makes its presence felt.
Winter is approaching so we must take courage, make the very best of the hand we've been dealt.

Week 31

October 17ᵗʰ 2020

PM announced three-tier plan, one medium alert, two - high, three very high. Levels to be imposed. Liverpool City area is tier three; can't mix indoors or in private gardens. Bars and pubs will be closed.

Gyms, leisure centres, betting shops, adult gaming centres, casinos were added to list of closures. People asked not to travel in and out of areas, but Whitty says tier three needs stricter measures.

Lancashire joins Liverpool in highest alert. Their move plus support of £42 million announced Friday. Soft play to close, not gyms and leisure centres. Leaders felt bullied by Downing Street; not happy.

It's tier 2 for Greater Manchester but move to tier three is expected. More negotiations on Monday. Tier two has no mixing of households indoors, in pubs, bars and other venues causing much dismay.

Most of Essex, York, Barrow in Furness, NE Derbyshire, Chesterfield, Elmbridge, Erewash and London Move from tier one to tier two, told Thursday. 28 million now in high tiers, over half the population.

Just under half the country is in tier one. Basic restrictions apply - masks, distancing and rule of six. Let's hope infection spread can be curbed and strict measures in high alert areas will produce a fix.

90% of Liverpool ICU beds are full. More patients in hospital than there were at start of first wave. Nightingale hospitals on standby in Manchester, Sunderland and Harrogate. The situation is grave.

Government set out to turn a 'tipping point' into a turning point but with tendency to befuddle. Changes and protracted negotiations with local leaders have made it a bit of a 'B----r's Muddle'.

Three Cs - avoid crowding, close contact, closed places. This week is about rules and yet more rules. N. Ireland bars, restaurants, beauticians and hairdressers closed for 4 weeks, two weeks for schools.

Nicola Sturgeon says Scotland in 'precarious' position but deaths aren't rising at same pace as spring. Wales is banning travellers from high-risk areas in UK. A short national lockdown they're considering.

25-year-old in U.S. is fifth person to contract Covid twice, second infection was worse than the first. Australian research finds SARS-CoV-2 lives up to 28 days if left in the dark. UV light kills coronavirus.

Curfew in Paris and 8 other cities, 9 pm to 6 am. Netherlands and Czech Republic in semi-lockdown. China tests 9m, an entire city's population. The UK isn't alone in its Covid-19 control breakdown.

Our 94 year-old Monarch made her first public appearance away from Windsor Castle for 7 months.
She visited scientists at Porton Down who dealt with Novichok attack and supported Covid response.

Looking lovely in pink, she unveiled a plaque in red-carpeted marque, Prince William at her side;
A wonderful smile after isolating for months. She's lucky to live in a castle, it's a good place to hide.

News is grim this week but nature knows nothing of that. Maple leaves turn red and beech to gold.
So let's enjoy our glorious autumn, struggle through winter to spring and do exactly what we're told.

Three-tier coronavirus alert levels.

Tier 1 – Medium Alert:

Meeting with others: Different households can mix indoors and outdoors in groups of up to 6. Must maintain social distancing from anyone not in your household.

Travel and transport: No restrictions but must wear a face covering. Avoid travel to tier 3 areas unless absolutely necessary.

Staying overnight: No restrictions on overnight stays but restricted to 6 outside household.

Going to work: Work from home where possible. Workplaces should be coronavirus secure.

Shops: All shops can open.

Hospitality: Restaurants, pubs, cafés and other hospitality venues can be open. They must close by 11 pm, last orders 10 pm and table service only.

Personal care: Hair, nail and beauty salons can open.

Exercise: Gyms, pools and leisure centres open.

Worship: Rule of 6 applies.

Weddings: Up to 15 people. Sit-down reception must be coronavirus secure.

Funerals: Up to 30 people at funeral, up to 15 at wake.

Care home visits: Visitors allowed from Tier 1 or with negative test.

Tier 2 – High Alert

Meeting with others: Groups of up to 6 can meet outside. Maintain social distancing.

Travel and transport: Can use transport but must wear face covering. Avoid travel to tier 3.

Staying overnight: Overnight stays only with household or support bubble.

Going to work: Work from home when possible. Workplaces must be Covid secure.

Shops: All shops can open.

Hospitality: Alcoholonly with substantial meal in pubs, bars and restaurants. Table service only.

Personal care: Hair, nail and beauty salons can open.

Worship: Open but households must not mix.

Weddings: Up to 15 for ceremony and Covid secure sit-down reception.

Funerals: Up to 30 for funeral and up to 15 for wake.

Care home visits: Indoor visits allowed with negative test. Outdoor visits allowed without test.

Tier 3 – Very High Alert

Meeting with others: Must only mix with household inside private homes and gardens. Can meet in public outdoor places such as parks and beaches but 'rule of 6' applies. Social distancing must be observed with people not in household.

Travel and transport: Travel restricted to shops, work and hospitality. Masks need to be worn. Travel out of area restricted to essential only.

Staying overnight: Can stay overnight only with household and not outside local area unless essential.

Shops: All shops are open.

Hospitality: Hospitality venues closed except for takeaway and delivery services.

Personal care: Hair, beauty and nail salons open.

Exercise: Gyms, pools and leisure facilities open.Indoor sports only with households.

Worship: Open but households must not mix.

Weddings: Up to 15 people can attend ceremony. No receptions allowed.

Funerals: Up to 30 people can attend funeral. 15 people can attend wake.

Care home visits: Negative test result needed to visit indoors but not outside.

Week 32
October 24ᵗʰ 2020

PM and Mayor of Greater Manchester, Andy Burnham, arguing over grant was this week's wrangle.
PM offered £60 million; Andy wanted £65 million. PM imposed move to tier three, sorted the tangle.

Barnsley, Rotherham, Doncaster and Sheffield in S. Yorkshire move to tier 3, fortunately undeterred.
Coventry, Slough and Stoke on Trent move to 2ⁿᵈ tier. By end of week, 7.8 m will be in highest alert.

Scotland to introduce new five-level alert system, tier 0 – 4. It will be introduced on November 2ⁿᵈ.
Alert system to last until virus wanes. Nicola Sturgeon warns a digital Christmas celebration beckons.

Wales introduced a 'Firebreak', almost complete lockdown on Friday. On November 9ᵗʰ it will end.
After half term, secondary schools will learn online for a week. Primary schools back after weekend.

Pupils isolating in 46% of secondary schools, 16% of primary schools, 400,000 pupils total, good few.
R number 1.2 to 1.4. Infections still rising but they're doubling every three weeks instead of two.

Death rate increases, Friday 224 deaths, 1000 hospital admissions, 20,530 cases of virus infection.
Spain is the first European country to reach a million cases. When will we have the vaccine injection?

Forty vaccines worldwide are in clinical trials, our Oxford vaccine is in advanced stages of testing.
Nine are in final stages, 240 in early stages. Encouraging, but with no vaccine date set, frustrating.

Test and Trace is only reaching 60% of contacts. They're failing to cope as cases increase in number.
Only 15.1% of test results within 24 hours. PM concedes that NHS Test and Trace must get better

£80 'Lamp' saliva test at Heathrow T2 and T5, results in under an hour, for places requiring a test.
Hong Kong accepted 'Lamp' test but other destinations insist on PCR test so no good for the rest.

'Human challenge' Covid trials start in January. Healthy volunteers to be infected in vaccine trials.
Government grant £33.6 million. Volunteers monitored round the clock; noses infected from phials.

90 UK sewage treatment sites test for coronavirus. It's an early warning system, looking for clusters.
Sewage trials tracked success in lockdown, low levels in summer then sudden spike in September.

Rishi makes changes to 'Job Support Scheme' to help businesses, hospitality and low paid workers.
Workers do minimum of 20% of hours, paid 66.67% of hours not worked, 5% covered by employers.

Covid symptoms study app tracks long Covid suffers. More likely if over 50, female and overweight.
More symptoms, not just a cough, at time of infection bring a greater chance of long Covid-19 fate.

Denmark, Maldives, Canary Islands and Mykonos join safe travel list. Lichtenstein has been removed.
Bookings for holidays in Maldives and Canary Islands soar. Our holiday options have just improved.

A cosy family Christmas looks unlikely for most with rule of six, unless you're in a big family bubble.
Children listening to Radio 4 told that Santa is a key worker so presents will be delivered no trouble.

Clocks change Saturday night, days will seem shorter, gardening time reduced, it will be dark for tea.
But we must remain cheerful, spring clean in winter, or look for better ways to keep ourselves busy.

Week 33
October 31ˢᵗ 2020

Five-tier system to curb virus starts in Scotland Monday 6 am. FM emphasises complying is urgent. 'We need to stick with it so let's keep doing it together and for each other,' says Nicola Sturgeon.

Most of Scotland is in tier 2 - travel, socializing, alcohol sales, wedding and funerals are all restricted. N. and S. Lanarkshire, central belt, Dundee tier three, 0 and 4 none, islands in tier one as predicted.

Fifth of England in tightest virus restrictions. Nottinghamshire and W. Yorkshire move to tier three. Warrington, Cheshire East move to tier two. REACT say 100,000 catch Covid each day, apparently.

SAGE critical of government. Says lockdown should be imposed now or hospital admissions will rise. Need to end 'Test and Trace' company and give it to local authorities as cases doubling every 9 days.

Alarming increase in Europe. Belgium goes into strict lockdown, health emergency, deaths are stark. France 600 cases in 100,000, Netherlands – 634, Belgium – 2,399. Czech field hospital built in Prague.

France starts 2nd lockdown after high daily deaths. Restaurants and bars close, schools stay open. Form to leave home for work, food or medical reasons, one hour exercise a day. Macron has spoken.

Germany closes bars and restaurants, gyms and cinemas. Pubs and restaurants close at 6 pm in Italy. Takeaways allowed. Gyms, cinemas, theatres close. Spain imposes curfew. It's in state of emergency.

AGILE, which tests new Covid-19 treatments, and Royal Liverpool University Hospital, test new drug. If given early, it may prevent hospital admission, Molnupiravir disrupts genetic makeup of virus bug.

12-minute Covid test will soon be available at 200 Boots stores. 97% accurate but costs 120 pounds. Private PCR tests needed for some destinations, cost anything from £129 to £220, or there around.

In REACT-2 study, 365,000 adults did a finger-prick test as an antibody test for Covid-19 infection. Showed antibodies drop quickly after infection, 26%. T-cells not tested; they could give protection.

Doesn't mean vaccine ineffective. Older adults have strong response to vaccine, side effects fewer. More antibodies present if intense exposure to virus, or continuous small doses as in health worker.

80% of hospital patients with Covid have low levels of vitamin D. D fights infections, 'flu and colds. Suggested everyone takes 10 micrograms each day this winter. It could help to boost low thresholds.

Sniffer dog trial to detect Covid goes to Paddington for trial among noisy and distracting railways.
Covid-19 positive volunteers are sent T-shirt and socks to wear and return after a couple of days.

NASA finds water on moon, dark side and bright. Artemis 111 landing of woman is planned for 2024.
'Moonshot' Covid tests put on ice. Earth's in trouble, must be time for trip to the moon to explore.

'Blustery' was BBC weather word of the week – blustery winds, blustery showers and they were right.
Shipping forecast exciting listening, gales and storm force 9. Dark gloomy days soon turning to night.

Hornby train sales rise 33% as people look for something to do and publishers see book sales soar.
Reading good choice, sitting comfortably in a chair, feet up, not lying down laying tracks on the floor.

NOVEMBER 2020

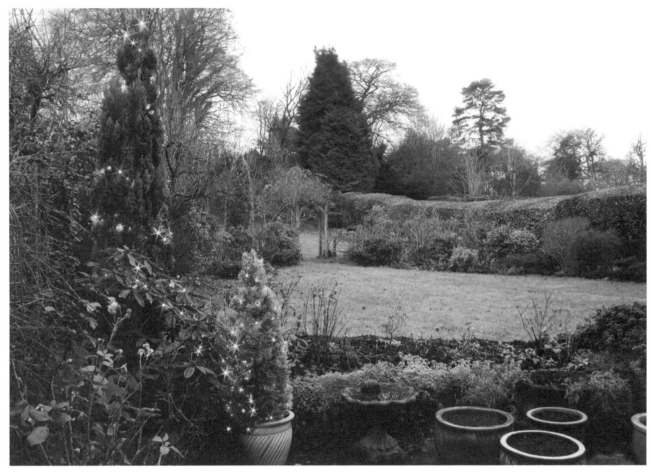

Christmas lights bring cheer to a November garden.

Week 34
November 7th 2020

Boris announced England's 2nd lockdown, less tight than March, from 5th November to 2nd December.
Still open are schools, universities, dentists, opticians, chiropractors, food shops and garden centres.

'Next slide, please, next slide, please' was Saturday night, Halloween, prime time TV entertainment.
Chris Whitty and Patrick Valance proved to us, with slides, lockdown was a necessary containment.

Allowed; meeting one friend on bench for snack, stay at hotel, exercise, work and visit to public loo.
Off limits; restaurants, pubs, leisure facilities, beauty salons, foreign travel, friends - to name a few.

Rishi Sunak extended furlough scheme until end of March, covers all UK nations, review in January.
Businesses get cash grants for forced closure. Furlough Scheme has cost 40 billion pounds already.

Day before lockdown was busy. Golf courses packed, Christmas shoppers flocking to shop in town.
Many enjoyed the sunshine on land and water, making the best of their freedom before lockdown.

Over 10,000 people in hospital. UK reached over one million cases of infection by beginning of week.
Deaths this week averaged 295 a day; almost 500 one day. Virus has spread quickly, outlook is bleak.

Covid cases are one in 90 in England, one in 110 in Scotland and Wales and, in N. Ireland, one in 75.
ONS data shows infections are stabilising, except in NE, and growth is levelling off, they derive.

Over 60,000 cases of Covid and 826 deaths in one day in France. 1.7 million Covid cases since start.
Greece started a lockdown for 3 weeks; Germany's ICU patients have doubled in 9 days. It's stark.

Germany and Sweden are back on the quarantine travel list. Free entry for Danish visitors is nulled.
Mink infected 200 in Denmark. In Jutland, there are 207 mink farms. 17m mink in 1,000 farms culled.

Mink found infected with Covid mutation in Spain, Denmark and Netherlands. Vaccine is threatened.
July 100,000 mink culled in Northern Spain. U.K. tourists brought virus back as borders untightened.

Closed Remembrance Service at Cenotaph Sunday. No march past this year, wreaths laid by royalty.
Public urged not to attend. Told to watch service on TV and observe 2 minutes silence in doorway.

Mass rapid Covid testing in Liverpool is offered from Friday, part of pilot, with frequent repeat tests.
Funding for marshals in England to encourage social distancing and mask use. A Covid security quest.

Lots of counting this week. Counting votes for US presidential election, then counting them all again. Counting DNA dissimilar Antarctic Gentoo penguins and counting days of lockdown that still remain.

Macchu Picchu opens after 7 months, only 700 visitors a day are allowed, not 5,000, but we can't go. So put exotic places on bucket list, dream of holidays for 2021. Plenty of time to save up the dough.

Bright days with frosty mornings herald the start of winter. Dahlias freeze and fuchsias shed blooms. There's tidying to do in the garden with falling leaves and lots of work with wheelbarrow and broom.

Week 35
November 14th 2020

Pfizer/BioNTech Covid vaccine caused great excitement, with some caution, around the world.
Gives 90% immunity to infection but may not prevent transmission. We must wait to be told.

RNA vaccine uses fragment of virus genetic material. Must be kept at -70C to -90C until last 48 hours.
GPs and pharmacies to roll out vaccination, maybe December, but the magnitude of this task towers.

UK ordered 40m doses in batches of 1,000. That will treat 20m as each person needs two doses.
Care home residents, care home workers, over 80s and health care workers will be the first focus.

Wales ends lockdown. Portugal in state of emergency, lockdown curfew 11 pm, 1 am at weekends.
Victoria, Australia, once centre of severe outbreak, has no cases of Covid or deaths as 4th day ends.

R number is now 1-1.2. Cases are falling in North West but rising in Midlands, South and in Wales.
50,000 deaths from virus in UK so far. 50 million cases of Covid worldwide and 10 million in the US.

Students will have 'lateral flow' test 3rd December. Test processed in an hour. If positive, a PCR test.
Must go home for Christmas by 9th December, but if positive, stay 10 days, then home for the fest.

Twenty care homes in Hampshire, Devon and Cornwall start Coronavirus testing trial next week.
One family member, or friend, will be tested, then allowed to visit resident in mask, so not idyllic.

Joe Biden's win, (Trump still doesn't concede), brings total change in presidential policies and style.
First priority is to control coronavirus. His task force will be led by private and public health officials.

Dominique Cummings, Boris' chief advisor, a controversial figure, quits, leaves Downing Street.
A maverick character and criticised for breaking lockdown rules. Finally, he makes a rapid retreat.

Diwali, Hindu Festival of Lights, started Thursday. Celebrations 'will be difficult' says Rishi Sunak.
People asked to meet virtually, light candles in windows and make sure lockdown rules are intact.

Queen's Platinum Jubilee, on 6th February 2022, will be celebrated with a 4-day holiday in June 2022.
By then, hopefully, we'll be vaccinated, can celebrate in style and happily hug and kiss everyone too.

John Lewis' Christmas advert is about kindness, inspired by public spirit during the virus pandemic.
Aldi's about loved ones reunited, Morrisons and Argos families at home, no need to be too dramatic.

We've all been affected by coronavirus somehow. Rupert Bear remains untouched as he turns 100.
Our anthropomorphic adventurer is honoured by Royal Mail in set of eight stamps with pullover red.

A wild, windy, wet weekend is expected. Walking and gardening will be on a 'between shower' basis.
But whatever the weather, news of the Pfizer/BioNTech vaccine will keep a wide smile on our faces.

Week 36
November 21st 2020

Good news this week. Moderna's RNA vaccine is on its way, can be stored at -20C. 30,000 in study.
95% effective and has been tested on vulnerable and elderly. Bad news is we haven't ordered any.

UK secures 5m doses for spring. US to roll-out vaccine soon. Million dollars gifted by Dolly Parton.
Pfizer applies to FDA for vaccine use and to regulators in UK, Europe, Australia, Canada and in Japan.

Pfizer/BioNTech says vaccine effective on all age groups and ethnicity with its 95% efficacy boost.
Matt Hancock says roll-out will begin next month if approved. At speed, vaccine can be produced.

Oxford vaccine shows 'encouraging' immune response in older adults. More data at end of year.
100 million doses on order for UK. Advantage is vaccine can be stored in normal refrigerator gear.

Russia's Sputnik V has registration certificate from Russian Ministry of Health. No one on trial fell ill.
Can be used to vaccinate population in Russia. Ongoing trials UAE, India, Venezuela, Egypt and Brazil.

Rheumatoid arthritis anti-inflammatory drug, Tocilizumab, seems to help critically ill patients in ICU.
Patients 87% more likely to improve than without it. Better than steroids. It may save quite a few.

Trial of AstraZeneca's jab for people without functioning immune system starts in Manchester today.
1,000 in trial. Uses antibodies from single US Covid patient. Could give at least 6 months' immunity.

Toughest restrictions in Scotland brought to 11 councils; includes Glasgow. 2.3 million in level four.
Restrictions to be lifted on 11th December. Only essential travel outside councils and that is law.

N. Ireland introduces tougher restrictions, start Friday 27th, only one week after lockdown lifted.
US has had 1/4M Covid deaths and 11m cases. It has suffered the most rapid spread in pandemic.

UK infections levelling off but hospital admissions still rising. Deaths topped at 529 on Wednesday.
Christmas celebrations for 1 day could mean 5 days of extra restrictions. Death is high price to pay.

Trial Covid test for relative or friend visiting residents in 20 care homes, Hants, Devon and Cornwall.
Matt Hancock says care homes to have testing for visitors by Christmas. Hopes to include them all.

It's been a bit of a comical week. PM pinged by 'NHS Test and Trace' to self-isolate along with 6 MPs.
Head of 'NHS Test and Trace', Dido Harding, pinged too. We have 10 more days lockdown until ease.

Beano comic has pull-out section to cheer adults – Boris and Cummings driving burglary getaway car. On way to Barnard Castle Cummings crashes, police ask about glasses, he claims contacts. OK so far.

Quebec school in red Covid area buys 3 wedding marquees. Moves pupils outside to reduce spread. Children love it. Good ventilation brings no cases of Covid. Congratulations go to innovative head.

All this vaccine talk makes us anxious for Covid-19 vaccinations to start. Life will be very different AC. Life BC was so easy, now it's WC, or 'With Covid'. We can't wait to welcome the vaccine with glee.

For now, we can only dream of meals out in restaurants, coffees in cafés, friends and being sociable. But one day our struggle will end. There'll be no need to wash our shop or try to dry the pineapple.

Week 37
November 28th 2020

New tiers bring tears of despair. Over 98% of the country is in tier two or three, the toughest tiers. Cornwall, Isles of Scilly, and Isle of Wight are tier 1. These lucky 700,000 can mix households indoors.

Tier 2 can meet in gardens,' rule of six', attend theatres, concerts and drink alcohol out with a meal. Kent and Bristol join Midlands, North West and East in tier three. Theirs a 'takeaway only' meal deal.

Last orders in restaurants and pubs 10pm, closing 11pm. Tier 3 can only meet in park with rule of six. Shops, gyms, hair salons, beauticians will open in all tiers. Next review 16th Dec., every two weeks.

Five days at Christmas, 23rd to 27th Dec, three households can bubble, meet indoors, but isolate first. PM says 'virus doesn't know it's Christmas'. Chris Whitty issues a 'don't hug elderly relatives' alert.

In Scotland, eight, not counting children, from three households can meet inside for Christmas span. Nicola Sturgeon advises them to wait until after they've been vaccinated to get together if they can.

Monday Oxford/AstraZeneca announced vaccine was 70% effective, 90% if first dose halved. Then, Thursday 62% effective. Half-dose with 90% efficacy was error. Trial was under 55s and only 3,000.

UK formally asked regulators, MHRA, to assess Oxford/AstraZeneca vaccine so progress is steady. Medicines and Healthcare products Regulatory Agency is reviewing Pfizer/BioNTech vaccine already.

R number falls, now 0.9.to 1. Infection curve is flattening but deaths are high - 695 on Wednesday. Infection rate elevated in secondary schools. 1 in 5 miss school, 22% of pupils were absent one day.

Coronavirus variant D arrived in UK on 29th January. By March it had mutated and become variant G. G variant of SARS-CoV-2 increases spread, more effective at entering cells so harder to become free.

Universities use lateral flow test 30thNov. 2 tests 3 days apart, if negative, go home with no delays. From 15th December, visitors can pay £65–£120 for test. If negative, shorten quarantine to five days.

'Our Health emergency is not yet over,' 'Our Economic emergency has only just begun'–- Rishi Sunak. Biggest slump in economy for 300 years, shrank 11.3%. Big rise in unemployment. Outlook is dark.

Biden's Covid team taskforce readies plan to fight virus. Cases now 13 million on increase path set. Trump pardons a Thanksgiving turkey; it's a tradition. There's talk he may even pardon himself yet.

Oxford English Dictionary can't choose just one word as 'Word of the Year' summing up a crazy year. Coronavirus, Covid-19, bubbles, social distancing, furlough, lockdown, all 2020 candidates it's clear.

In 2020, sales of both dogs and cats went up, for amusement at home, to love or take out for a walk. Temperatures plummet making gardening unattractive. Better to keep busy with a knife and fork.

DECEMBER 2020

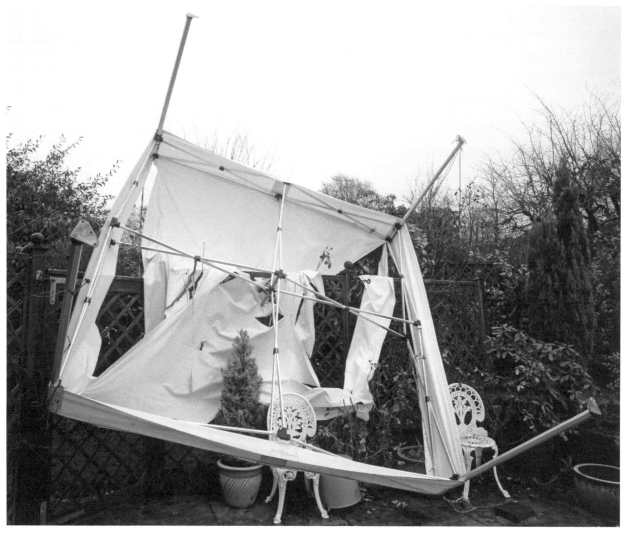

Gazebo wrecked by storm Bella on Boxing Day. It sums up our feelings for 2020.

Week 38
December 5th 2020

'The needle has landed' – Sun. Vaccine's arrival in UK as momentous as Apollo Eagle moon landing. MHRA passed Pfizer vaccine on Wednesday. Vaccine arrived by Eurostar from Belgium next evening.

Pfizer vaccine transported in dry ice 'thermoboxes', Pfizer's design, lasts 10 days if box unopened. 5 days max in fridge. 'It's not a yoghurt that can be taken in and out of the fridge,' warns Van-Tam.

800,000 doses will be distributed to 50 hospitals from hub. Vaccination to be rolled out next week. Difficult to deliver to care homes as vaccine unstable. Order of 9 priority groups may need a tweak.

Over 80s and elderly in hospitals will be given vaccine, then NHS workers, but care homes must wait. GP conglomerates start vaccinating 14th December, will be sent 975 doses. 80+ then as doses dictate.

Hospital Trust is working on ways to split batches for rollout. Splitting batches is MHRA approved. Care homes need small batches as can't store. Now they'll have vaccine in 2 weeks; problem solved.

Rolling out the vaccine is a mammoth task, speed essential with 975 doses in each batch to use fast. Cranleigh's village hall has been approved for distribution. Need ways to distribute vaccine full blast.

UK bought 2 million more doses of Moderna vaccine. Applied to EUA as vaccine clearance it strives. Nadhim Zahawi appointed Minister in charge of Covid-19 vaccine rollout. He commits to saving lives.

Infection rates in England fell by 30% in lockdown; now they're 1 in 105. Death rates alarm and stun. Infections one in 185 in Wales, one in 145 in N. Ireland, one in 115 Scotland. R rate is now below 1.

In Wales hospitals are struggling, NHS at breaking point. Severe restrictions introduced on Friday. Pubs, restaurants and cafés can't sell alcohol, must close at 6 pm. Can't travel to tier 3, 1 and 2 only.

US has over 280,000 deaths but fewer than UK per million, Spain and Italy more per million than UK. UK reaches 60,000 deaths to Covid-19, nearly one in 100,000. Need effective vaccine without delay.

Biden, Obama, Bush and Clinton pledge to be vaccinated on TV. To boost public confidence the aim. Polls in US indicate many are reluctant to get the jab. Facebook removes every false vaccine claim.

Government introduces 24-hour opening for all shops and eleven Primark stores will do just that. Vaccine arrives. Thundersnow hits Scotland. Booms like an explosion as snow extends thunderclap.

George Eustice told LBC radio Scotch eggs are a meal. 10 pints of beer and a scotch egg if you please.
He said they were a substantial meal if served at a table. Michael Gove told LBC radio he disagrees.

Marquees, tents and patio heaters spring up outside pubs. Is winter eating outdoors such a doddle?
Pubs advise wearing thick clothes. Say 'bring your own and they'll be happy to fill a hot water bottle'.

Japan drops asteroid rocks by parachute in Australia which may reveal origins of life on Earth untold.
China puts a flag on the moon, collects rocks from 'Ocean of Storms'. Oh, what an astonishing world.

Week 39

December 12th 2020

6.31am Tuesday – Maggie, first in world outside trials, receives Covid-19 vaccine in Coventry hospital.
Maggie, 91 next week, said it was the 'best early birthday present' – our light at the end of a tunnel.

Over 80s in hospital and visiting outpatients received jab Tuesday. Excess vaccine went to NHS staff.
Cards are issued with vaccine type, batch number and the date of the second jab for the other half.

Pfizer vaccine has 50% efficacy with first dose. 2nd dose after 21 days, 95% immunity after a week.
Two had adverse reaction. If 'significant history of allergic reaction', an alternative it's wise to seek.

Matt Hancock said it was 'historic moment' and dubbed Tuesday 'V Day'. Not sprint but marathon.
There are 3.2 million over 80, 25 million in vulnerable groups over 50. The queue will go on and on.

From Monday, Covid vaccination programme, CVP, for GPs begins but only small amount is available.
Gradually it will be rolled out to 1,000 GP groups. In 2021 a greater vaccine rollout will be attainable.

Canadian regulators have passed the Pfizer vaccine. FDA, US regulator, at last, passed it yesterday.
Lancet Journal publishes Oxford trial results. 70% efficacy and may prevent transmission they say.

New trial planned for January, one dose of Pfizer and one of Oxford vaccine, best of both worlds.
Combination of Sputnik V and Oxford vaccine trials will start in Russia. New approach this heralds.

Russia rolls out Sputnik V to population but many sceptics stay away as they're uncertain of data.
China's Sinovac Covid-19 vaccine 'CoronaVac' is in final stages, worldwide orders organized for later.

In Wales, Covid cases surge; could be third wave. 400 more in hospital in December than in April.
Neath Port Talbot nearly 700 cases in 100,000. Schools close Monday, cases have reached high level.

US deaths nearly 300,000. California is in lockdown for 3 weeks, stay at home order for 85% of state.
With ban on mixing households, many businesses close. Thanksgiving celebration sealed their fate.

German and S. Korean cases rise. Bleak situation in Sweden with 99% of beds taken in Stockholm.
ONS survey says cases in UK 13% down. In some areas, they've risen but in others, they've fallen.

London, Kent and Essex have elevated level of virus, particularly among secondary school children.
Home online lessons, mass testing to identify cases, drop before Christmas hopefully put in motion.

Eleven councils in Scotland move out of level 4. Glasgow, Lanarkshire, Renfrewshire to name a few. Pubs must serve food, alcohol takeaway only. Non-essential shops open, pubs and restaurants too.

Canary Islands are put on UK quarantine list. Self-isolating reduced from 14 to 10 days across UK. Covid negative test after 5 days can half isolation. Travellers could still enjoy Christmas if they pay.

Genetic makeup is proven to affect Covid infection severity. Genomes of ICU patients mapped. Faulty TYK2 gene causes immune system to overreact, inflammation results and body is entrapped.

Christmas card messages this year start with 'what a year', or similar. We've had a topsy-turvy year. Jammy Dodgers are displayed heart and raspberry jam side downwards in packet. In chaos, it's clear.

Week 40
December 19th 2020

130,000 Pfizer vaccinations were rolled out in the first week of vaccination programme in England.
Town halls, churches, even racecourses and football grounds used for vaccination schedule planned.

Vaccination of residents in Welsh and Scottish care homes started. England to follow soon they say.
975 vaccine doses divided into 195 x 5 vials can be transported frozen and stored undiluted 5 days.

Moderna/NIAID vaccine, 94% efficacy, and Oxford/BioNTech vaccines still await authorization in UK.
Pfizer vaccine now being rolled out in US. Moderna vaccine approved for use in US with no delay.

Mike Pence, VP of the US, receives Pfizer vaccination on TV to boost confidence and safety promote.
Emmanuel Macron tested positive for Covid-19 prompting several European leaders to self-isolate.

London is moved into tier 3, top tier, Cambridgeshire, Buckinghamshire, Berkshire, Hertfordshire and
Bedfordshire, most of Surrey, parts of E. Sussex and Hampshire move too. 38 million in tier 3 band.

Pubs and restaurants closed except for takeaway, mixing households allowed in public places alone.
Bristol and N. Somerset move down to tier 2, Herefordshire joins Cornwall and Isle of Wight in tier 1.

US now has 3,000 deaths a day. Washington's Cathedral bell tolls 300 times for 300,000+ lives lost.
Germany locks down for Christmas, 950 deaths in 24 hours, schools, restaurants, businesses closed.

Netherlands and Italy are in lockdown. France curfew 22.00-06.00, form to leave home is needed.
New outbreak in Sydney, Australia. Residents told to stay at home; travel to other states impeded.

Ireland starts 6-week lockdown on Boxing Day, Wales starts lockdown on December 28th, so bleak.
Boris is 'hoping to avoid' lockdown, R number rises 1.1 to 1.2 with 660,000 infections in one week.

New Covid-19 mutation in over 1,000 cases in S.E. UK, scientists start work on what this could mean.
They're trying to establish if the rapid spread in S. England is linked to changes in the 'spike' protein.

Boris warns small, short Christmases are safer Christmases. Elderly should meet only after vaccine.
Chris Whitty says 'keep it small, keep it short and keep it local'. A plea to let good sense intervene.

Scotland advises cutting Christmas to 1 or 2 days. Five days is opportunity, not a recommended time.
Welsh FM, Mr Drakeford, cuts 3 household Christmas bubble to 2. Made law, breaking it is a crime.

Staggered return for pupils in January. Only exam years will return to school at the normal time. Secondary pupils to be tested before returning to school, until then, teaching carried out online.

Parish of Dedham and Ardleigh in N. Essex plans 'Drive-In Carols' in farmer's field with fun routine. Cars parked using social distancing, streamed service on the radio, a gospel choir and a giant screen.

UK is manufacturing solar-powered vaccine freezers to be exported to Nigeria which is good news. Sales of scotch eggs have rocketed, up 100%, pubs are selling them as a main meal to go with booze.

Christmas presents will arrive as usual on Christmas Eve. Santa will work as normal in community. Exempt from travel restrictions, he'll fill good children's stockings. All reindeer have herd immunity.

PM added a 4ᵗʰ tier to Tier Alert System 19ᵗʰ December 2020

Tier 4 – Stay at Home

Stay at home:	Only leave home for essential food shopping, medicines, work, education, exercise, medical care.
Meeting with others:	Only members of household can meet indoors and in garden. Can only meet one other person in public place. Must maintain social distancing.
Travel and transport:	Cannot travel out of area unless essential. Face covering.
Work:	Must work from home if possible.
Shops:	Non-essential shops closed. Food and essential shops open.
Hospitality:	Hospitality venues closed apart from for takeaways.
Personal care:	Hair, nail and beauty salons closed.
Exercise:	Indoor gyms, pools, leisure facilities closed. Outdoor facilities open.
Worship:	Can stay open but cannot mix outside households.
Weddings:	Limit of 6 in exceptional circumstances.
Funerals:	Up to 30 people.
Care home visits:	Outdoor, at windows or in specially designed Covid secure room.
Christmas:	No Christmas bubble. No households can mix indoors or in garden.

For Christmas Day alone, tiers 1, 2 and 3 can form a bubble with up to 2 other households indoors.

Week 41
December 26th 2020.

We've passed the darkest day of the year, 21st, passed Christmas with its joy and disappointments.
A turkey for 10 was shared, if you were lucky, but in new tier 4, eaten alone with no extra recipients.

On Boxing Day 6 million joined the top tier 18 million. 43% of the country is in top tier, new tier four.
Suffolk, Oxfordshire, Norfolk, Cambridgeshire, Essex, E. and W. Sussex must tier four now endure.

Joining London, Kent, Buckinghamshire, Berkshire, Hertfordshire, Essex, Surrey already T4 imposed,
They have a stay at home order. Non-essential shops, indoor pools, hairdressers and gyms all closed.

Travel out of tier four is forbidden. Only one person can meet one person in public place like a park.
Schools stay open and you can go to work but otherwise tier four looks a lot like lockdown - stark.

Northern Ireland and Wales are in lockdown and Scotland in level four, very close to lockdown too.
UK deaths reach 70,000. More people in hospital now than there were at peak of first wave. It's true.

The new Covid-19 variant is highly transmissible. It's spreading across UK and threatening Europe.
France closed border to UK Monday. 5,000 lorries stuck in Kent; M20 is in a nose-to-tail back up.

Over 50 countries banned UK arrivals, most European countries, US, Canada, Russia and even China
But new variant is in Netherlands, Sweden, Denmark, Germany, Italy, Switzerland, Japan and Austria.

France demanded Covid testing, 15,000 tested with 36 positive results, border opened Wednesday.
Many spent Christmas in their lorries. Asked to rate M20 on Trip Advisor if they enjoyed their stay☺

Another new variant found in S. Africa, even more easily transmitted. UK put restrictions on arrivals.
If arrived from S. Africa in last 14 days you must self-isolate along with any close contacts, it's radical.

Covid reaches Antarctica, 36 Chileans fall ill. 26 army and 10 maintenance workers at research base,
Evacuated to Punta Arenas. Now Antarctica, last Covid-free continent, in pandemic has a place.

Oxford vaccine has all the data and is looking for authorization. It could be authorized by Thursday.
Pfizer/BioNTech has finally been authorized in Europe and vaccination started after annoying delay.

500,000 in UK have had Pfizer vaccine but Jeremy Hunt said no more supplies till March - no slack.
Pfizer said all was progressing according to agreed schedule. Vaccine arrives early 2021, 'on track'.

New monoclonal drug trial started by University College Hospital, to be AstraZeneca-manufactured.
10 people given drug, an injection of antibodies. It's used as quick treatment if Covid-19 factored.

100mph gusts and flooding as Storm Bella wreaks Christmas havoc. Pub marquees and tents beware.
Fallen trees, houses flooded with 5 feet of water. For some this was 'Worst Noel' ever, a nightmare.

Flour and pasta already restricted in Tesco. Now eggs, rice, toilet rolls, hand wash numbers capped.
Brexit is sorted and prices for food won't rise, so they say. A Christmas present for all - gift-wrapped.

Queen in Christmas speech, all people want 'for Christmas is a simple hug or a squeeze of the hand'.
'Even on the darkest night, there is hope in the new dawn' brought comfort to our troubled land.

JANUARY 2021

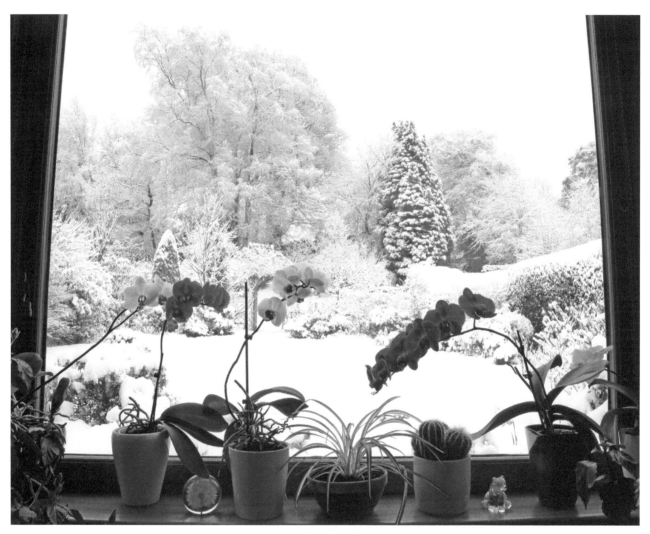

Warmer inside than out.

Week 42
January 2nd 2021

'NHS' and 'Hope Together' lit up the night sky as 2021 was ushered in to an eerily quiet London city.
Giant blue bird created with drones hovered over O2 Arena with fireworks filling the sky, very pretty.

10 million watched laser light displays, drones and fireworks on BBC 1 TV as they set the sky on fire.
Scotland's Hogmanay was celebrated with drones forming images of galloping stag and Saltire.

Promise of a better year dawned. Vaccine 'Oxford's Christmas present to the world' Sarah Gilbert.
AstraZeneca's vaccine authorised early in week has given UK vaccination plan much needed support.

Over 80s' vaccination starts Monday in earnest. In Scotland, 80+ vaccination starts 11th January.
12-wk interval for Pfizer vaccination approved but a wait until spring for Moderna vaccine delivery.

Jab with 2nd jab in 12 weeks debateable. Vaccine shortage and virus variant surge changed itinerary.
BioNTech says 1st jab prevents serious illness, larger gap before booster jab gives greater efficacy.

Government claims supply of vaccines responsible for delay in rollout. Manufacturers disagree.
They claim supply is in compliance with schedule agreed with government, not a lack of capacity.
Most second vaccinations after Monday are cancelled but GPs told they can use clinical discretion.
Disputers claim vulnerable betrayed and lack of testing of long interval between Pfizer vaccinations.

Argentina has approved AstraZeneca and Pfizer vaccines and started with Sputnik V from Russia.
Brazil hasn't approved any vaccines but, with rising cases and deaths, is being put under pressure.

UK Tuesday 53,135 new cases, Thursday 55,892, Saturday 57,725, in hospital 20,436, a record.
UK deaths in 24 hours 981, in U.S. 3,923 and in Brazil 1,200. Deaths across the globe have soared.
Most of Leicester, Lincolnshire, Nottinghamshire, Derbyshire, Warwickshire, Gloucestershire,
Staffordshire, Lancashire, Cheshire, Cumbria, Somerset and Greater Manchester move to top tier.

78% of the country is now in tier 4, most of the rest in tier 3. Isles of Scilly only remains in tier one.
New variant hugely transmissible, leading to 60% of infections. UK is 'back in the eye of the storm'.

Mutated virus found in Colorado man who hadn't travelled. Variants are now dangerous runaways.
200 tourists fled Verbier by night after tourists and skiers from UK told to quarantine for 10 days.

Secondary school return delayed. 11th Jan exam years, rest 18th back, mass testing before return.
Primary schools start 4th January, except London schools where all learning must be done at home.

Police broke up numerous large, illegal parties on New Year's Eve making arrests and issuing fines.
Hospitals are facing 'tsunami' of Covid cases, likely to increase after partying on these massive lines.

Over 200 Pandemic volunteers and professionals were honoured in the New Year's Honours list.
Lewis Hamilton was knighted for achievements in motor sport and seven F1 driver championships.

It's been a week of contrasts, good and bad, with vaccines bringing hope but virus variant spiking.
We just need to wait patiently, follow all the rules, until the vaccine ticking clock starts striking.

Week 43
January 9th 2021

Monday PM announced 3rd lockdown from Wednesday. Stay at home, schools and colleges closed.
Work at home, essential shopping only, exercising with household or just one friend is unopposed.

Mainland Scotland and Isle of Skye stay at home order from Tuesday, schools closed until February.
Wales have extended lockdown three weeks. Lockdown restrictions throughout UK are necessary.

Schools open for keyworkers' children and those without space to work at home or electronic aids.
'A' levels, GCSEs and National exams in UK will not go ahead this summer; teachers to select grades.

537,000 doses of AstraZeneca vaccine are available, deliveries begun, but rollout is slow, uncertain.
Churchill Hospital started Oxford vaccine batch 0001 on Monday, 7.30. Vaccinated 82-year-old Brian.

PM's aim is to vaccinate 14 million by 15th February, frontline health, care workers and all over 70s.
Only 1.5m vaccinated so far so ramp-up planned. Armed forces will help with battlefield strategies.

Seven mass vaccine hubs set up in; Excel Centre London, Millennium Point Birmingham. Stevenage,
Epsom Race Course Surrey, Newcastle, Bristol, and Manchester. Huge project and hard to manage.

223 hospitals, 700 local and 180 GP led sites roll out vaccine. No one need travel more than 10 miles.
200 pharmacies will take part in pilot scheme with major Boots and Superdrug stores to stock vials.

RNA Moderna vaccine cleared for UK use. Part of virus genetic code stimulates immune responses.
Has nearly 95% efficacy, but no deliveries until spring. UK increased order from 7 to 17 million doses.

Race between infection and injection. Variant is 50-70% more transmissible and accelerating fast.
30,370 in hospital, 1,041 deaths Wednesday, 1,162 Thursday and 1,325 Friday, a record, angst vast.

On Friday, London Mayor declared major incident. Cases one in 20-30, 35% higher than in last April.
Virus 'out of control'. Firemen and police to drive ambulances. 7000 with Covid admitted to hospital.

Government has new slogan - 'Act like you've got the virus' - unpleasant concept, and could depress.
Each of us must take responsibility for spread of virus but 'Keep yourself safe' would depress us less.

Anti-inflammatory drugs, Tocilizumab and Sarilumab, can now save quarter of sickest patients in ICU.
£1,000 a patient but used in conjunction with cheaper drug dexamethasone speeds up recovery too.

Covid test up to 72 hours prior to departure for UK arrivals, countries without infrastructure exempt.
Quarantine for arrivals 10 days unless country on safe travel list. A £500 fine for avoidance attempt.

Clapping for NHS staff and carers returns on Thursdays. It's been renamed 'Clapping for Heroes'.
Muted response, enthusiasm has waned, or is it that coldness and darkness indolence has imposed?

Prince William talked on Zoom with London hospital medical staff. Asked how they were coping.
Expressing thanks and voicing support for their hard work, he showed concern and understanding.

For now, we must keep cheerful. Not let freezing fog, sheet ice and snowfall add to our Covid woes.
Home workers who cleared John Lewis stores of own brand slippers are happy with their toasty toes.

Week 44
January 16th 2021

3.2 million have received a first dose of the vaccine, some the second, but it's a postcode lottery.
90% of 80s+ vaccinated in Cheltenham, national average 36.5%, rollout in some areas a mockery.

130,000 over 80s have been sent vaccination invitations, 600,000 more will be receiving one soon,
Appointments booked online, available seven days a week. We're working on becoming immune.

Six high street pharmacies became vaccination centres. 200 more will provide jabs in next 2 weeks.
Must be able to give 1,000 jabs per week and have space to social distance; some will need a tweak.

EasyJet's crews are being trained to deliver vaccine. Reaching 15m jabs by Feb 15th will be a hassle.
Queen (94) and Duke (99) waited their turn and were vaccinated on Saturday in Windsor Castle.

AstraZeneca is increasing production from 1.1 million doses to 2 million a week. Production is fast.
Pfizer is making plant improvements. 'Short-term' impact on supplies to UK but delay won't last.

36,797 Covid cases in hospital, twice as high as at peak in April. Hospitals are getting ready to burst.
Wednesday 1,563 deaths, a record. Over 88,575 deaths total. More deaths in 2nd wave than in first.

Scotland tightens lockdown rules. Takeaways only from hatch, essential items for click and collect.
Workers only allowed indoors for maintenance. No drinking in public places with immediate effect.

'Next few weeks are going to be the worst', said Chris Whitty, as sadly the coming days will prove.
'It is always darkest just before the day dawneth' T. Fuller (1650), gets worse before things improve.

Cases are plateauing in some parts of the country with R number 0.9 to 1.2. A welcome 20% drop.
Lockdown is working, but deaths for 7-10 days will be at their worst as holiday season deaths top.

Survey showed 83% immunity after infection for at least 5 mths, although some reinfections arose.
Reinfections mild but could infect others. This is what the survey with 20,000 health workers shows.

Lateral flow testing prioritising factory, shop and front-line workers across the country will go ahead.
Idea is to use rapid tests to identify infections, particularly asymptomatic cases, to stop the spread.

Tesco, Sainsbury's, Waitrose and Asda will challenge those without masks. Some will forbid entry.
In Wales, Covid measures for shops are made law. Numbers restricted so shops must get ready.

New Brazilian variant brings concern. May interfere with antibody effectiveness which is alarming,
Ban on travellers from Brazil, S. America, Portugal and Cape Verde is in place from Friday morning.

All travel corridors will close 4am Monday to prevent virus variants from entering and last sometime.
Arrivals need negative test result, must now quarantine 10 days. After 5 days released if 2nd test fine.

Supreme Court rules business interruption policies with insurance companies valid, liability is found.
Tens of thousands of small businesses to get insurance payouts worth 100s of millions of pounds.

Sun and sand summer bookings soar. Over 50s are hoping for vaccination with jabs round the clock.
Puffer jackets are selling like hot cakes. Cosy, comforting coats are needed for walk round the block.

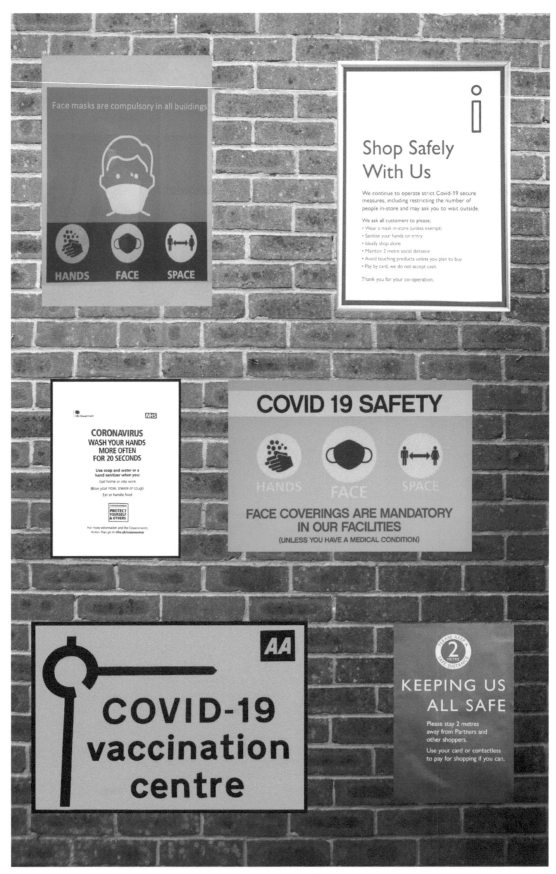

Signs and posters displayed during pandemic

Week 45
January 23rd 2021

In UK, 200 vaccinations are being given every minute. Now a first dose has been given to 5.4 million. 65 more vaccination centres have opened, a cinema in Aylesbury and a mosque in Birmingham.

Vaccine delivery is 'lumpy'. 2/3 of 80+ vaccinated in Yorkshire and NW, ½ in London and South East. Supplies to some centres being cut to make rollout more even will help others get started at least.

5 ½ million invitations for vaccinations have been sent out to areas where 80s already vaccinated. Over 70s and the extremely vulnerable invited. Disparity across country leaves over 80s frustrated.

Ten more mass vaccination centres open, including Taunton Racecourse and Blackburn Cathedral. R number lower, between 0.8 and 1. New virus variant may be 10–50% more deadly than original.

39,000+ in hospital with Covid. Some ICU nurses, caring for 5 patients, not 1, are care time bereft. Patients are admitted to hospital every 30 seconds. Many hospitals have no critical care beds left.

ONS found infections doubled between October and December. Antibody tests were planned. Antibodies found in 1 in 12 in N. Ireland, 1 in 11 in Scotland, 1 in 10 in Wales and 1 in 8 in England.

Tuesday 1,610 deaths and Wednesday 1,820, the biggest daily figure since the pandemic started. A total of 95,000 deaths. UK is close to first in record deaths per million that are Covid-19 related.

India has its first 'injection of hope'. BioNTech and Covaccines used on population of 1.3 billion. 3,000 centres are set up to vaccinate 100 a day. By end of July, the plan is to inoculate 300 million.

Joe Biden, the 46th President, says vaccine rollout a 'dismal failure'. He promises a wartime strategy. US deaths reached 400,000. He intends to ramp up vaccine production, vaccinations, tests and PPE.

Biden re-joins WHO, will support COVAX in working for global equitable access to Covid-19 vaccines. COVAX will accelerate manufacture of vaccine. UK has given ½ billion to this very worthy scheme.

Germany mandates medical-grade masks in workplace, shops and on public transport, N95 or FFP2. Austria and France set to follow Germany. The UK is considering changing mask-wearing advice too.

Covid sufferers recovering at home are given oximeters by hospitals to report readings to GPs daily. If oxygen level drops below 94%, it could indicate serious complications which could turn deadly.

N. Ireland lockdown extended until March 5th. Storm Christoph flooded AstraZeneca store in Wales.
Glastonbury is cancelled in June for the second year. There's a drop across England in clothing sales.

A wedding with 150 guests was broken up by police. Organizers fined £10,000 with £200 for guests.
Next week, party of 15 or over will mean fines of £10,000 for organizers and £800 each for the rest.

Hospitality told they may not be able to open again until May was met with shock and dismay.
Saga says only those vaccinated welcome on their cruises which are due to start at end of May.

Snowdrops, daffodils and hellebore herald approach of spring, longer days will help spirits restore.
90-year-old man said getting vaccinated was best thing to happen to him since the end of the war.

Week 46
January 30th 2021

Almost a year to the day since coronavirus was first detected Covid deaths in the UK passed 100,000.
Grim milestone with UK deaths worst in the world and tragic year of loss, our hearts are saddened.

30% of Covid-19 deaths occurred in care homes. Like wildfire, the infection spread at a terrible cost.
PM said 'I take full responsibility for everything the government has done' and is sorry for lives lost.

R number is 0.7 to 1.1. Infection rates are falling over most of country but levels are still far too high.
Mid-Feb we'll know if vaccinations are preventing hospitalizations and changes it could then justify.

Lifting lockdown depends on vaccination progress, deaths and hospitalization. That's PM's format.
Lockdown will continue until at least 8th of March and schools won't return any time before that.

But Welsh primary schools may return after half term if infections continue to fall with no peaks.
Scotland's lockdown won't finish before mid-Feb. Wales has extended their lockdown by 3 weeks.

UK citizens arriving home from high-risk areas must isolate in hotels for 10 days and meet expense.
S. Africa and Brazil are on 'red list' as their new variants of the virus threaten our vaccines' defence.

8.4 million in UK have received their first dose of vaccine. On track for our 15th Feb 15 million target.
EU authorized use of Oxford/AstraZeneca vaccine but say UK must meet any shortfall in market.

AstraZeneca's two vaccine plants in Europe have ongoing problems and can't work to full capacity.
Can supply only quarter of EU needs and wants UK supplies. UK's contract with EU under scrutiny.

Moderna vaccine effective for UK and Brazilian variant but may not be as effective against S. African.
Moderna to make new variant booster shots but not until spring are any supplies for UK in the plan.

Sanofi, French drug company in Frankfurt, is to manufacture Pfizer vaccine from July to boost supply.
Sanofi to produce 125m doses to help Pfizer as it is struggling with the huge demand it must satisfy.

Novavax, US biotech company, to produce vaccine in Stockton-on-Tees. It's in stage 3 trials in UK.
89.3 % efficacy, 83% against UK variant, 60% against S. African. UK's 60 m doses for April underway.

Janssen, in Belgium, owned by Johnson & Johnson, has a vaccine 66% effective with only one dose.
85% effective in preventing severe disease after 28 days. Application for MHRA approval is close.

English National Opera to work with 1,000 people with long Covid to improve breathing and anxiety.
Second-hand books snapped up as backdrop for Zoom calls to give appearance of being scholarly.

Snowfall across UK delighted children this week and turned the landscape to sparkling white jewels.
Two students fined £10,000 each for organizing snowball fight in Leeds which broke lockdown rules.

Now the snow has melted and temperatures risen, we see signs of spring once again in our gardens;
Yellow crocus and fragrant Daphne bloom as winter retreats and nature our gloominess pardons.

FEBRUARY 2021

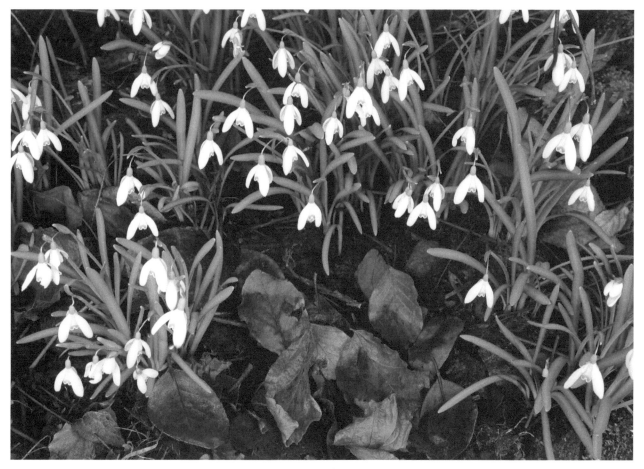

Snowdrops

Week 47

February 6th 2021.

Captain Sir Tom died of Covid on Tuesday. He raised 33m for NHS and inspired others to accomplish. He gave us a lift when we needed it with a cheeky twinkle in his eye. He was the very best of British.

The second wave has peaked, R number fallen, is 0.7 to 1, but infections are still high, substantial. One in 60 has virus but deaths have decreased by 10% and fewer are being admitted to hospital.

11 cases with S. African E484K mutation have no link to travel so variant is spreading in community. In total, 105 cases found and identified in postcodes W7, N17, WS2, ME15, PR9, EN10, GU21, CR3.

80.000 over 16s will be tested. PCR tests delivered door to door and collected an hour or two later. Mobile testing units in some areas will test for positive cases to add to the collection of new data.

S. African variant may make vaccines less effective. Plan is to produce updated vaccines by autumn. RNA vaccines are easier to tweak but all vaccines must be updated to cope with evolving mutations.

15th February all arrivals from 33 countries on 'red list' will have to quarantine in hotels for 10 days. 1,450 arrivals a day are expected from S. America, Portugal, UAE and most South African countries.

11m have had first dose of vaccine, 85% uptake. BAME communities mostly are the 15% refusals. 98% care home residents, 90% over 75s done, 50+ by May to be vaccinated and clinically vulnerable.

39 more vaccination centres opened this week, including 2 theatres and Basingstoke Fire station. Also, Crystal Palace football ground's hospitality lounge and Debenhams empty store in Folkestone.

UK has ordered 407m vaccine doses. Could give one dose to everyone 6 times with different brands. UK has ordered 100m doses of Valneva, a French vaccine, to be produced in Livingston, Scotland.

Research shows Oxford vaccine has 76% efficacy 3 mths after first shot. 2nd dose increases it to 82%. Vaccine significantly reduces transmission, is effective against Kent variant so is fine for the present.

Germany, France, Poland and Italy are advising against giving AstraZeneca vaccine to the over 65s. Switzerland hasn't placed orders for AZ vaccine as it's waiting for new data from studies and trials.

There's concern second Pfizer vaccine dose is needed sooner than 12 weeks to protect the elderly.
Antibodies from one dose are not sufficient and serious illness could occur through lack of immunity.

Trial with 820 volunteers starts next week with one dose of AstraZeneca and one of Pfizer vaccine.
Could help with disruption in supply and may give broader protection. In June, results will be seen.

Russia plans trial with one dose of Sputnik V and one of AstraZeneca in the hope it will raise efficacy.
Sputnik V is 91.6% effective. 15 countries have approved it including Argentina, UAE and Hungary.

Olympics will take place in Japan this year with restrictions. You can't sing, chant or cheer, only clap.
Masks essential except eating, sleeping or performing outdoors. Masks shouldn't create a handicap.

Vaccine rollout is like a bright rainbow cutting through the dark clouds in a heavy shower of rain.
Our hope is when the rain stops and the dark clouds clear the sun will shine and all will be well again.

Week 48

February 13th 2021.

England's vaccine rollout has been great success. 14m vaccinated, on track for 15m on 15th February. Wales reached target 12th Feb. Scotland on track. Pfizer vaccine supply low but dip only temporary.

Over 65s to get invitations for vaccinations from Monday 15th. Rollout speed varies across country. Some centres at only 5-10% capacity, reasons under review. Possibly ahead in the group delivery.

Monday arrivals from 'red list' must quarantine for 10 days in hotel booked online at cost of £1,750. Online payment includes cost of transport and tests. Two PCR tests on 2nd and 8th day, rules abound.

Fine for failure to quarantine in designated hotel £5,000-£10,000. 4,700 rooms in 16 hotels reserved. False travel history reported on mandatory passenger locator could see 10 years in prison served.

Guests can go outside with staff for fresh air. Scotland will quarantine all overseas arrivals in hotel. In England, other arrivals must quarantine 10 days at home, have 2 PCR tests, costing £210 as well.

S. African strain B.1.351 with E484K mutation able to dodge antibodies. For immunity this is salient. S. African study of 2000 showed AZ vaccine didn't prevent mild or moderate infection from variant.

Prof. Van-Tam said that S. African variant wasn't a major threat in UK as it wasn't spreading quickly. Urged people to get vaccinated. WHO said go ahead with vaccine. It would be some help anyway.

Oxford/AstraZeneca is working on booster for S. African variant. It will be ready for use in autumn. Early results from studies show Pfizer and Moderna give more protection against a variant problem.

R number is 0.7-0.9. One in 80 has virus in England, one in 85 in Wales and one in 120 in Scotland. Infections shrinking by 2%-5% every day but numbers still very high. The Kent variant is dominant.

Director of Covid-19 genomics UK, Prof. Sharon Peacock, said Kent variant had 'swept the country', Would probably 'sweep the world'. Kent variant in over 50 countries. A worry in Australia already.

Trials of steroid dexamethasone with arthritis drug tocilizumab found to keep patients from ICU, Reduce Covid-19 deaths of those needing oxygen by 1/3 and of those requiring ventilation by ½ too.

Boris is expected to announce road map for lockdown ease in the week starting 22nd February. Masks and social distancing may stay until autumn. We're not likely to get back to normal anyway.

£125 billion has accumulated in people's bank accounts over lockdown, ready for a spending spree.
With the economy shrinking by 9.9% during 2020, the same certainly isn't true of the economy.

Government accused of sowing confusion about booking summer holidays. Can we or can't we go?
Grant Shapps said 'Don't book holidays for home or abroad' as it's far too early to know.

So, avoid disappointment, book a holiday somewhere you don't like then you can cancel with ease.
Lovely blue skies but it's freezing cold. Braemar, Scotland, recorded temperature of -23C degrees.

Texan lawyer appeared as wide-eyed fluffy cat in virtual court hearing. Cat tried to explain in vain.
Video went viral, brought levity to pandemic Zoom-fatigued world, was played over and over again.

Week 49
February 20th 2021

Sunday 14th Feb PM announced 15 million people had been vaccinated with one dose. Target met. He thanked those who had played a part. A target to get all over 50s vaccinated by end of April set.

Aim is to give all second doses within 12 weeks. 3,000-4,000 second doses are being given per day. Manchester mass vaccination centre has many free slots. It's a preference for local centres they say.

Boris chaired G7 meeting. He encouraged all richer countries to give surplus vaccines to the poorer. 'Until we're all safe, no one is safe'. While virus is continuing to circulate, it will mutate still further.

Monday PM will present 'roadmap' for easing lockdown, to be done gradually as caution dictates. PM and Scottish FM want to work in parallel to lift lockdown. Plan to be governed by data, not dates.

Care home residents can pick one person to visit them regularly from March 8th, can hold hands. Visitors must wear PPE and take test before visit. Lockdown ease to include outdoor meeting plans.

Scottish primary schools return Monday 22nd. Secondary top 3 years if course has practical element. Welsh 3-7-year-olds on Monday. Return of older pupils will be number of covid-19 cases dependent.

AstraZeneca vaccine trial for 6 – 17-year age group to start. 300 volunteers near 4 hospitals sought, In Oxford, London, Southampton and Bristol. 240 to receive AZ and 60 a meningitis jab, it's thought.

England to start Covid human challenge trial; is recruiting 90 volunteers. Ages 18 to 30 are eligible, Must be in good health, paid £4,500, monitored for year and will stay 17 days in Royal Free Hospital.

It's the first human Covid-19 trial in the world. Low dose of the live original virus given in nasal spray. Object of trial to see level of virus needed to cause infection. A vaccine trial will later get underway.

Surge testing for South African virus variant is expanding to Southampton SO15 and Norfolk IP22; Positive cases will be sequenced for genomic data to understand variant and spread of virus too.

Infection rates have been dropping across UK, down by a half but still high. 553,000 now affected. In August it was 250,000 and mid-January 1,250,000. Still over 25,000 in hospital with Covid infected.

1 in 115 in England, 1 in 180 Scotland, 1 in 125 Wales and 1 in 105 Ireland have the virus at present. R number is down 0.6–0.9. 41% of over 80s have antibodies, 15.7% overall in UK, an increase of 3%.

Airborne transmission has become a concern and is being monitored. Better masks may be needed.
Some countries insist on N95 masks being worn on public transport so that entry of virus is impeded.

1.7m letters are being sent out to extend the clinically vulnerable advised to shield, now 4 million.
Chronic illness, weight, ethnicity are factors. They'll be prioritised for vaccine under new definition.

6ft 2in, 32-year-old man was offered vaccine in a priority category so he phoned his GP as uncertain.
17 stone, height 6.2cm, BMI 28,000, he was morbidly obese. It's a basic algorithmic computation.

We're all walking on the same bits of grass and paths for exercise and now it's all puddles and mud.
Advice is to wear wellies. Don't walk where wildflowers grow. Go straight through mud and flood.

Week 50
February 27th 2021

PM presented his' roadmap', a long route to freedom. Data must be achieved before arrival 21 June.
Bit like a fairy story. The prince has to slay a dragon before he can claim his princess and her fortune.

Freedom is still months away. Schools return 8th March. Enjoy coffee on a park bench with a friend.
March 29th 6 can meet outdoors, or 2 households. Outdoor sports open. Stay at home order to end.

It's 5 weeks before step 2 on April 12th. Pubs and restaurants can serve meals and alcohol outdoors.
Non-essential shops, holiday lets, zoos, theme parks open, personal care & hairdressers – applause!

Step 3, 17th May, maybe. Sports events open, indoor venues of 1,000, outdoor up to 4,000 people.
Indoor hospitality, indoor exercise opens. Life events such as weddings up to 30 guests may mingle.

Step 4, 21st June, we hope. Legal limits on social contact removed, nightclubs reopen, time to party.
Steps by data; vaccine rollout, effectiveness, new variants, NHS coping will all influence guarantee.

Scotland's lifting of lockdown to be 'cautious, sure and steady' using tier system. No end date given.
Phase change is every 3 weeks. All in tier three by last week of April. Opening is to be safety-driven.

Covid alert level lowered from highest level of 5 to 4 as the risk of overwhelming NHS has receded.
Hospital admissions high but manageable, 1100 a day, down from peak when 4,000 was exceeded.

GCSE and A-level results to be set by teachers, combination of mock exams, course work and tests;
No algorithms so difficult to standardise. Results will be 2 weeks early to facilitate appeal requests.

Queen took part in video call with health leaders. She said vaccine 'quite harmless, didn't hurt at all'.
Virus is ' bit like a plague, it's everywhere'. 'Keep up the good work,' she said with a smile to enthral.

'It's difficult for some people.' 'Should think about other people rather than themselves,' she said.
11-15% vaccine-hesitant. Many in ethnic minority groups. Hopefully they can be by our monarch led.

29% of population vaccinated in UK, 91% in Israel, 59% in UAE, 20% US, 6.8% in Germany, very few.
'Liebe Briten. We beneiden you!' Front page of Germany's Bild Newspaper. 'UK, We envy you'.

UK deaths 122,415 but falling daily. Infection 7-day average 8,500. R number 0.6 – 0.9 in England.
Infections are one in 155 in England, 1 in 195 in N. Ireland, 1 in 205 in Wales and 1 in 225 in Scotland.

15th April vaccinations move to third stage. Keyworkers won't be prioritised. It will go by age solely.
40-49-year-olds group 10, next group 30-39, then 18 to 39. Everyone vaccinated by the end of July.

Vaccine passport, do we, or don't we? Israel has app on phone to prove person has been vaccinated.
It's needed for entrance to synagogues, hotels and leisure centres. Shops open to all, not regulated.

Spring is on its way literally and metaphorically. 'The crocus of hope is poking through the frost',
Said PM in his address on easing lockdown. But nature's spring is sure with no threat it might be lost.

Cat called' Storm' brought live pigeon to a virtual Stormont meeting, much to the owner's chagrin.
To show it was unhurt, he cradled the bird in front of camera. The owner's name was Colin Pigeon.

MARCH 2021

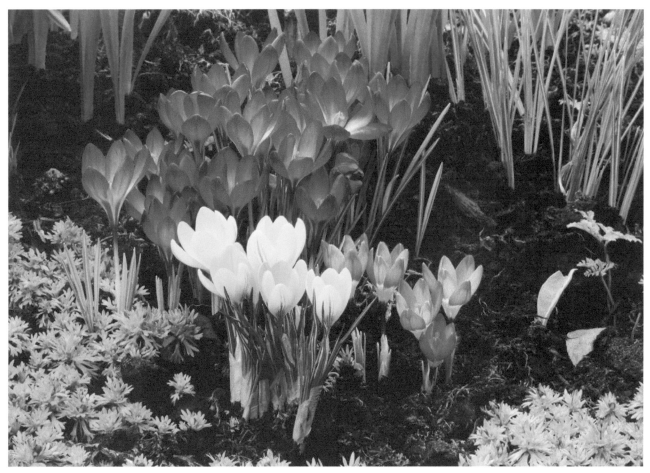

Purple and yellow crocuses.

Week 51
March 6th 2021

Monday, schools go back. Schools to test secondary pupils 3 times, then tests twice weekly at home.
To reduce aerosols, open top windows is advice. Secondary school mask use puts them on their own.

Over 21m have had first dose of vaccine, 1m second. 60-63-year-olds sent vaccine invitation letters.
Now 1,800 vaccination sites in England. Community pharmacies will be added to the other centres.

Present vaccine supply will double by the 15th March. Vaccine supply is now lower than it has been.
Prof. Sarah Gilbert is awarded the Royal Society of Arts Albert Medal for work on Oxford/ AZ vaccine.

Vaccines effective in saving lives of over 80s, reduced serious illness 80% and reduced transmission.
1 in 24 in England has antibodies, one in 8 in Scotland, one in 6 in Wales and N. Ireland, in addition.

Italy has stopped 250,000 doses of AstraZeneca being sent to Australia, much to Australia's dismay.
Australia uses Pfizer, has received 300,000 doses of AZ, will produce own from mid-March, so okay.

Studies show 90% of deaths from Covid in countries where over 50% of population is overweight.
'Clear and compelling correlation between obesity and death from Covid', ten times the death rate.

New variant is added to UK watch list of 8. 16 cases of new UK variant found with E484K mutation.
6 cases of Brazilian variant found in England and Scotland. Mystery case traced to Croydon location.

Infection rates across the country dropped a third in a week but drop slowed or has risen in places.
In England 1 in 220, Wales 1 in 285, N. Ireland 1 in 325, Scotland 1 in 335, progressively fewer cases.

EU is to adopt vaccine passports, to be known as 'Green cards'. Need smart phone to display app.
Include test results if not vaccinated. UK 'working with international partners on issue,' said Matt.

Cyprus to welcome tourists from UK a week after they've had both jabs, from the beginning of May.
Earliest anyone can go abroad on holiday is May 17th. Portugal joins Cyprus as it feels the same way.

Isle of Man introduces 21-day circuit-breaker, new spike of 60+ cases, some are of unknown origin.
Most were the result of one ferry worker infected in UK. Full lockdown on Wednesday has come in.

Cancer and inflammatory arthritis sufferers, immunosuppressed, in collaborative university project.
Those with impaired immune system vaccinated to see how much immunity is produced to protect.

Efforts being made to contact those who haven't been vaccinated; must persuade them it matters.
Ghana President vaccinated with AstraZeneca under COVAX scheme on TV to help encourage others.

Before Dolly Parton had her Moderna shot, she sang 'Vaccine, vaccine, vaccine' in her Jolene rewrite.
'I'm begging you not to hesitate. Vaccine, vaccine, vaccine. Once you're dead that's a bit too late'.

Dolly gave 1m dollars to develop Moderna vaccine. She encourages vaccination with all she's got.
Smiling she says 'All of you cowards, don't be such a chicken squat. Get out there and get your shot'.

Winter is fading as snowdrops, crocuses, primroses and daffodils push up through dry, dead leaves.
And as the vaccine rolls out across the globe each citizen vaccinated a massive sigh of relief heaves.

Week 52
March 13ᵗʰ 2021

Greece and Spain welcome UK tourists with negative test results, antibodies or proof of vaccination.
France opens its borders to tourists with negative Covid-19 test, becomes another travel destination.

EU countries have level of infection 3 times greater than UK, apart from Spain which is doing well.
Italy, Poland, Hungary and Czech Republic have rising Covid cases. Czech cases very high, no parallel.

Where it's possible to travel to and return from without quarantine at present is very hard to tell.
Grant Shapps, transport minister, says it's too early to book anywhere, wait until report 12ᵗʰ April.

10 cases of Brazil variant, P.1. in UK, 3 more in S. Gloucestershire and one from Brazil in Bradford.
US study finds Pfizer vaccine effective against P.1. AZ says prevention from serious illness is secured.

Norway, Denmark and Iceland have suspended use of AstraZeneca vaccine. Denmark for 14 days.
No evidence AZ vaccine responsible for blood clots causing alarm. 30 cases in 5m, so a survey says.

Over 23 million have received first dose of Coronavirus vaccine in UK. Nearly 1.5 million second dose.
Vaccine supply increased; one plant boosted output 50%. July target for all adults vaccinated is close.

AstraZeneca vaccine can produce a reaction, fever, headaches, sickness and fatigue after first dose.
Pfizer produces less of a reaction after first but a bigger reaction after second dose, a study shows.

Biden eyes 4ᵗʰ July as 'Independence Day' from virus. On track to vaccinate all eligible by 1ˢᵗ of May.
Johnson and Johnson to provide 100m single-dose shots by end of March and deliver without delay.

Infections in England and Wales fell last week overall, although they are rising in S. West and S. East.
R number is 0.6-0.8, a 30% drop in infection since last week. Number of deaths is much decreased.

Sewers are playing a part in identifying areas where virus is present giving early warning of infection.
Samples taken every hour from wastewater are sent to labs for analysis and mutation identification.

Researchers identify inflammatory protein, Cytokine called GM-CSF, linked to severe Covid-19.
Increase in GM-CSF in early stages of infection indicates those who will be critically ill or die it seems.

Scotland 4 people from 2 different households can meet outdoors including gardens from Friday.
Four 12-17 yr olds can meet from 4 different households. 26ᵗʰ March places of worship open to pray.

Wales lifts stay at home order, advice is to stay local, within a 5 mile radius. Hairdressers can reopen.
Most non-essential shops closed till April 12, phased opening. Garden centres March 22 will open.

Some outdoor sports may reopen. 4 people can meet from 2 households outdoors including garden.
Care home visits will restart for single designated visitor. Primary schools and exam years to return.

3 million new pets acquired by families, couples and singles to increase company during pandemic.
Out of all the animals chosen, dogs are most popular, 2.3 million added to households for friendship.

The pandemic has brought many a change in our daily lives and in our vocabulary too, of course.
The game played by young boys of ringing doorbells then running away is renamed 'Parcel Force'.

Week 53
March 20th 2021

Oxford/AstraZeneca vaccine, used and manufactured all over the world, is not without its troubles.
13 EU countries, 17 countries in total, suspended use. Vaccine schedules became an utter shambles.

Blood clots, including rare clots in central vein in brain, reported amongst those newly vaccinated.
UK cases men, EU young women. Germany 13 with 3 fatalities. Review starts to see if AZ related.

European Medicines Agency, WHO and MHRA announced later in the week benefits outweigh risks.
France, Germany, Spain and Italy resumed AZ use. Netherlands and Portugal wait till Monday to fix.

France won't give AZ to anyone younger than 55. Denmark, Sweden and Finland are still thinking.
Germany may use Sputnik V when licensed. Delay in vaccination costs lives people could be living.

In UK, 26.7m first vaccine doses given, ½ adult population, but supplies for April suffer sudden glitch.
1.7m doses of AZ held to test stability. 5m doses from India delayed. Their own need causes hitch.

Texts have been sent to 2m in the 50–54-year age group, encouraged to book vaccine appointments.
Deaths from Covid in over 80s fell 86% in March. Vaccination has provided steady improvements.

Infections in France are rising. S. African variant is a major concern and should be taken seriously.
EU cases soar. Italy plans total Easter lockdown and in Germany, cases are growing exponentially.

First lockdown anniversary is March 23rd. Boris says he's sorry he didn't introduce lockdown earlier.
UK highest death rate in Europe, fifth highest in world, but our vaccine rollout is happily superior.

UK deaths have now reached 126,026. It's a sobering total, highlighting need to get vaccinated.
Hartlepool GP surgery received 126,000 calls the day after news of poor supply. People irritated.

Scotland to lift stay at home order 2nd April; must stay within local authority until April 26th though.
Hairdressers and garden centres open April 5th. Pubs, restaurants, gyms April 26th get green to go.

England waits until 17th May for hospitality and gyms to open as well as gatherings for life events.
In Scotland, two households can meet indoors from 17th so no longer they'll be shivering in tents.

Holidays in Europe at present are threatened. Bookings in June, July and August discouraged.
High infection and slow vaccination progress in Europe could cause rise in UK if travel mismanaged.

BA will recognize proof of two vaccinations on app. Turkey open for tourists without vaccine records.
P&O plans 2 British Isles cruises. Twice vaccinated are eligible a week after 2nd vaccination onwards.

Dominic Cummings said Health Department was 'smoking ruin' when pandemic in March struck.
Trip to Barnard Castle to test eyesight makes him well able to recognize ruins; his record has stuck.

We've had some beautiful sunshine this week although a NE wind has brought a keen chill to the air.
Spring flowers fill gardens and as lockdown is still in place there's ample time to just stand and stare.

Week 54
March 27th 2021

Tuesday named 'Day of Reflection'. It marked the passing of one year since start of first lockdown.
At midday, a minute's silence to think of those who died of Covid-19 as pandemic year came around.

At 8 pm candles were lit at front doors and torches beamed into sky as a beacon of remembrance.
One in 500 of population died. Major landmarks bathed in yellow light proclaimed tribute in silence.

Vaccination will end pandemic but 'None of us is safe until all of us are safe', UN Secretary-General.
Serum Institute in India is largest AstraZeneca vaccine producer in the world. Their role is essential.

But India is holding back supplies. UK has vaccinated over 30m with 1st dose and 3m with second.
27m second doses must be given and more first doses too. It's all about a reliable supply in the end.

EU row with UK over vaccine supply with veiled threats continues. Now looking for win-win solution.
Europe with only 12% of population vaccinated, is desperate for vaccine supply as in a dire situation.

Much of Europe has third Covid-19 wave and France has increasing infections of S. African variant.
PM says spread will inevitably 'wash up on our shores' and vaccines not S. African variant resistant.

While spread of virus increasing the chance of new dangerous mutations occurring is more likely,
Vaccine given per 100 people, 44.7 UK, 37.2 US, 12.9 EU, 5.7 Russia and 5.2 China. UK world envy.

Booster jab to protect against newer variants could come as early as September for the vulnerable.
Nadhim Zahawi says there'll be 8 vaccines by autumn and a one-shot vaccine for 3 variants available.

US authorized AstraZeneca vaccine. 76% effective, 86% for over 65s and 100% against serious illness.
It took them a while and they complained about out-of-date data but finally they declared it riskless.

Backlash from hospitality. PM suggested vaccination proof may be needed for a pint and pub entries.
UK may wait till all adults offered vaccination. Vaccine passports are proceeding in other countries.

Fines of £5,000 have been introduced for anyone trying to leave the UK without a good reason.
France is put on UK's red list of 37 countries. Arrivals must stay in a hotel for 10 days to quarantine.

Fall in Covid cases mainly levelling off but in Scotland rising slightly. R number in England 0.7-0.9.
Friday 6,187 UK Covid cases, 70 died. Rise of infections in secondary schools but primaries are fine.

ONS found 1 in 10 died 6mths after release from hospital, 1 in 3 readmitted, 1 in 20 had heart attack.
Trial using Atorvastatin, statin, and Apixaban, blood-thinner, hopefully, will keep recovery on track.

Wales is first to have stay at home and stay local order lifted. Caravan parks and campsites open.
Self-contained accommodation available only for Welsh to holiday, not for all UK a holiday option.

11 yr old Max Woosey raised £270,000 by sleeping in his garden in a tent for a year; deserves praise.
North Devon Hospice funding was down due to Covid and they'd cared for his friend in his final days.

On Monday, stay at home order lifts in England, can drive somewhere, have party for 6 in garden.
Forecast for sunshine, Spanish temperatures, clocks changed. Party time at last, that's for certain.

APRIL 2021

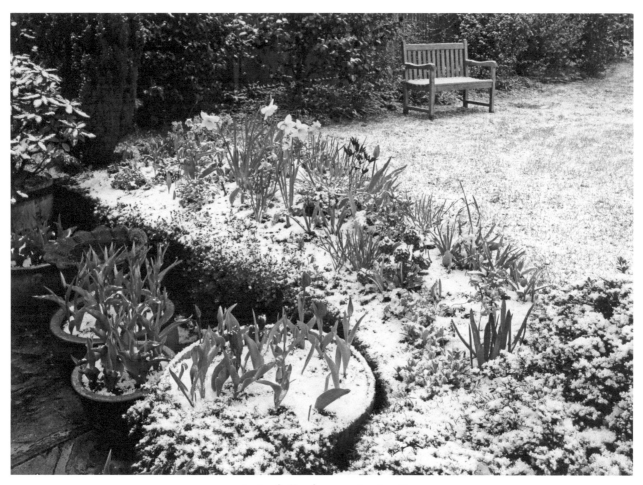

Late fall of snow in April

Week 55
April 3rd 2021

Freedom to entertain in the garden combined with the arrival of high temperatures was perfect.
For the very lucky ones, gazebos were erected in gardens full of spring flowers and guests expected.

On 30th, highest temperatures in March for 53 years were recorded, 24.5 C, 76.1F in Kew Gardens.
There was punting on the Cam, full parks in London and on beaches people amassed in their dozens.

April will be vaccine's second dose month as 12 weeks comes around for all those vaccinated first.
31.3 million first doses given and 5 million of second. UK is very definitely vaccination focused.

Lenny Henry and black celebrities signed a letter urging black communities to take vaccine offered.
Ethnic take-up low, 58.8% black African, 68.7% black Caribbean. For whites a 91.3% take-up assured.

Novavax manufactured in Teesside by Fujifilm will be bottled by GlaxoSmithKline in Barnard Castle.
UK ordered 60 million doses of Novavax. Has 100 million vaccine doses surplus to give away in total.

Moderna vaccine will arrive in UK soon. Wales and Scotland begin next week giving Moderna shots.
France, Germany, Holland and Canada use AstraZeneca only for over 60s. Say risk of rare brain clots.

In February more than 1m people had long Covid in UK. Middle-aged women, 35-49, worst affected.
Suffering from breathlessness, fatigue, muscle pain and brain fog for long after they were infected.

France, Italy and Germany are battling a third wave. New European vaccine plants will open directly.
AstraZeneca in Leiden, Netherlands, Moderna in Basel, Switzerland and Pfizer in Marburg, Germany.

Travel ban for people travelling from Pakistan, Bangladesh, Kenya and Philippines is from Friday.
Nationals, Irish and residents arriving must quarantine in government-approved hotels for 10 days.

Royal Caribbean Cruises are sailing from Southampton round the British Isles providing staycations.
Proof of first and second dose of vaccine will be essential when booking your British waters vacation.

12 countries on green list for travel from May 17th may include UAE, Malta, US, Portugal and Canada.
'Planes to Spain fly mainly to Bahrain.' Spain 11% vaccinated, Bahrain 33%. Vaccine clinches agenda.

In Scotland, people can meet in gardens and parks for the first time as stay at home rule is lifted.
But they must stay local, not move between authorities for three weeks, leaving many frustrated.

Introduction of vaccine passports is dividing opinion. Some say they'd be divisive and discriminatory.
QR code on smartphones is already in use in New York. Boris will tell us about UK plans on Monday.

60% of pubs won't open on April 12th. No outside space, or too little, makes opening unprofitable.
Two households, or a group of six, can sit outside for a meal, or even to just enjoy a drink is possible.

Pfizer vaccine given to 2,260 12-15-year-olds in a US study was found to be 100% effective.
Pfizer is seeking FDA authorization for use in US. To seek MHRA approval in UK is an objective.

Salisbury Cathedral used as vaccination centre. Organist played relaxing music to extend hospitality.
300 hours he played as 25,000 vaccinations took place. Album will be released to fund NHS charity.

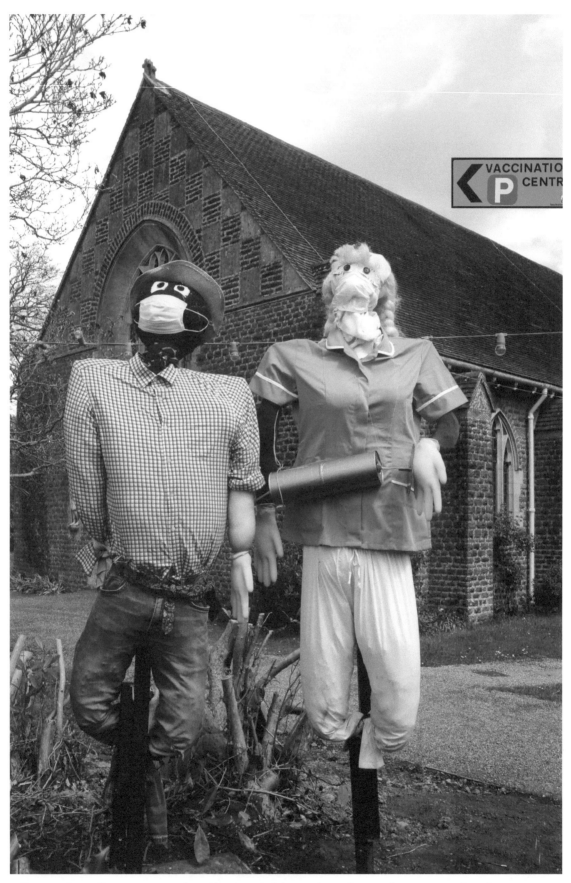

Dummies of a nurse and patient outside a church used as a vaccination centre.

Week 56
April 10th 2021

People are no longer being advised against booking foreign travel so book now if travel is a passion.
All travellers must take a PCR Covid test costing £120 before travelling and another on their return.

A list of countries marked with a traffic light system will be announced at the beginning of May.
Green no need to quarantine. Amber quarantine 10 days at home. Red 10-day approved hotel stay.

Jet2 has suspended flights until at least June 23rd as so much uncertainty in government travel plans.
Guernsey won't welcome any visitors until 1st July so visitors must wait if they're Channel Island fans.

Two free lateral flow tests are now available to everyone from pharmacies, test centres or by post.
Discussions continue as to whether PCRs could be made cheaper or LFTs used for travel uppermost.

April 12th will be an exciting day for many. Non-essential shops can stay open until 10 pm at night.
Hairdressers open from 8-10 pm 7 days a week. Now women's crowning glory will at last be all right.

Pubs can serve food and drinks outdoors to parties of 6 or 2 households, there are still rules to obey.
Gyms, self-catering accommodation, campsites, zoos, personal care, libraries all open from Monday.

First UK Moderna shots were given on Wednesday in Carmarthen in Wales and Glasgow, Scotland.
Three vaccines available in UK will help with supply. Next week Moderna jabs will roll out in England.

MHRA and JCVI reviewed the link between Oxford/AstraZeneca vaccine and very rare blood clots.
79 cases in UK, 51 women, 28 men, with 19 deaths. Three deaths were in the under 30-year-old slot.

They decided benefits still outweigh risks but there is a link and risks should be listed as a side effect.
Headaches, shortness of breath, swelling of legs, chest pain, blurred vision never should we neglect.

UK will not give AstraZeneca to under 30-year-olds. They will be given the Pfizer or Moderna vaccine.
Many countries will restrict AZ to older age groups. A problem with Janssen vaccine is also foreseen.

UK infection rates have fallen. Friday 3,150 compared to 6,397 a week ago. R rate in England 0.8 - 1.
Covid deaths now fallen over 92%,1,006 in one day at January peak to 40 deaths Saturday, a fraction.

Vaccination is bringing down infections. 26m first shots and 6m second given in total by end of week.
1 in 350 infected England, 1 in 300 N. Ireland, 1 in 410 Scotland, 1 in 800 Wales, lower than at peak.

In Brazil cases are soaring, over 4,000 deaths a day, 348,934 in total, caused by virulent P.1. strain.
President downplayed seriousness of virus, resisted lockdown, use of masks and use of any vaccine.

Saturday, India had 145,000 infections and 800 deaths, attributed to reluctance to wear a mask.
India's 'double mutant' strain has 2 mutations that bind to cells increasing urgency of vaccine task.

UK is saddened by the death of Prince Philip. He's been praised for devotion to country and Queen.
During the pandemic, 'HMS Bubble' was created for Prince Philip, a few staff and our own Sovereign.

It's been cold this week with snow in the south on Tuesday and low temperatures bringing frost.
But flowers, once buried in snow, raise their heads high again as spring continues and all is not lost.

Week 57
April 17ᵗʰ 2021

Prince Philip's funeral, low key and in line with lockdown rules, was Saturday in St George's Chapel. Masks worn, only choir of four sang, social distancing observed and there were 30 guests in total.

Prince Philip's coffin in a green open Land Rover, his own design, was followed by family walking. Queen arrived in State Bentley and sat alone. Royal vault was Prince Philip's final place of resting.

Monday shoppers flocked to high streets. At 6 am, some hairdressers set about tidying DIY haircuts. It was very chilly but holidays still began for many in boats, caravans, tents, cottages and even huts.

Scotland's ban on travel beyond area lifted and six from different households able to meet outside. Welsh shops and hairdressers have opened but opening of pubs before 26ᵗʰ April they'll be denied

Northern Ireland stay at home order lifted after 3 months but told to work from home and stay local. 23ʳᵈ April hairdressers open and on April 30ᵗʰ outdoor hospitality, gyms and all shops non-essential.

Surge testing is tracking S. African variant B.1.351, with E484K mutation, in 6 councils in S. London. 56 new cases were found in Wandsworth and Lambeth this week. Now 600 in total across nation.

Indian variant, B.1.617, with two spike protein mutations that help it infect cells, has arrived in UK. Dangerous as it evades immune system. 73 cases in England and 4 in Scotland found to UK's dismay.

Indian infections surge to well over 200,000 a day, possibly caused by the 'double mutation' variant. Brazil has many 30-50-year-olds in ICU. P.1 virus variant's aggressive and deadly properties salient.

Denmark has fully withdrawn use of AstraZeneca vaccine over blood clots affecting one in 40,000. Risk of clotting 10 times greater from Covid-19 than it is from AZ. That's what UK recent trial found.

All adults on Fair Isle, UK's most remote island community, vaccinated with two doses of AZ, no less. J & J pauses rollout of Janssen in US, Europe and S. Africa; blood clots in young women, one death.

Moderna rolls out in England. Effective against S. African variant but immune response isn't strong. UK vaccine advisers say pregnant women should be offered Pfizer or Moderna vaccine before long.

By Tuesday, over 50s had been offered vaccine ahead of April 15ᵗʰ target. Over 45s can book online. 32.7 million first doses have been given and 9.1 million have had first dose and the second on time.

Com-Cov calls for volunteers over 50 who have had one dose in last 12 weeks for mixed vaccine trial. Same vaccine or Moderna or Novavax given. Efficacy is monitored, could change vaccination style.

ONS finds Covid-19 infections have fallen in a week. 180,000 cases fell to 130,000, a drop of 28 %. But variants, South African and Indian, are a concern. Focus is now on all new dangerous variants.

Gardens have been important in lockdown, not only for fresh air and a place we're allowed to meet. Gnomes gained popularity. Now there's a national shortage of gnomes, stone, plastic and concrete.

Week 58

April 24th 2021

On Radio 4, leading scientist, Sir Jeremy Farrar said Covid-19 is now endemic, no longer a pandemic. Diagnostic tests, genomic sequencing, treatments, vaccines help control infection as it gets sporadic.

ONS survey of 370,000 found all age groups after one vaccine dose are 65% less likely to be infected. 90% less likely after two doses of Pfizer. AstraZeneca's 2nd dose results to come later but expected.

There's been a 95% uptake of vaccine in the over 50s but only 80% in care home staff in community. Pfizer boss says people will need third dose between 6 and 12 months after 2nd to retain immunity.

March Covid-19 was no longer leading cause of death in England and Wales, first time since October. Number in hospital has fallen to under 2,000. Friday, new deaths 40, new cases 2,678, getting lower.

Surge testing for S. African variant extended to Birmingham - Tile Cross, Alum Rock and Glebe Farm. Cases of S. African variant B1351 increases 5.5% to 644. It's the variant that can do the most harm.

55 new cases of Indian 'double mutation' variant detected. B.1.617 infections now total 132 in UK. India is put on UK red travel list. Arrivals had to quarantine in designated hotels from 4 am on Friday.

Infections in India have soared. 330,000 in one day with 2,300 deaths. The situation in India is grim. Six hospitals in Delhi have no oxygen and all ICU beds are full. Any chance of quick control now slim.

Large cities in Brazil are badly affected by virus, hospital ICU beds 90% full, variant highly contagious. Coronavac, Chinese vaccine, and AZ used. 11% 1st dose, 4% 2nd. Pfizer refusal earlier was outrageous.

China has had only 4,636 deaths from Covid-19. For months they've eaten in restaurants and cafés. Borders remain closed. Four Chinese vaccines and being vigilant have helped the Covid-19 squeeze.

COVAX programme which supplies vaccine to developing countries now 90 million doses in arrears. India's Serum Institute is prioritizing India for AZ produced. COVAX is looking for doses from S. Korea.

Gyms and non-essential shops in Scotland open Monday. Pubs and restaurants can serve outside. Wales brought changes forward. Indoor activities open 4th May, hospitality open May 17th inside.

Wall Street Journal reported first fake Pfizer vaccines found by cyber police in Mexico and Poland. 50 took part in Germany's vaccine tours to Russia for Sputnik V vaccine as rollout very slow at home.

PM said 'Antiviral Task Force' has been set up to run trials on new drugs to stop Covid in its tracks.
Trials of a pill taken at home when positive test or members of household fall sick with Covid attack.

New generation of vaccines likely to be nasal sprays or tablets. In future, they'd become the norm.
!3 companies in US are working on a nasal spray vaccine and 5 companies on vaccine in tablet form.

Oxford University human challenge seeks 64 18-30-year-olds who've had Covid. Must be volunteers.
Trial to see the lowest dose causing infection; if ill, given antibodies to avert serious infection fears.

Domino's Pizza reports record sales in 2020 and 2021. It plans more outlets as Covid-19 fuels sales.
There's a shortage of packets of tomato ketchup as takeaways so popular, Heinz ketchup bewails.

MAY 2021

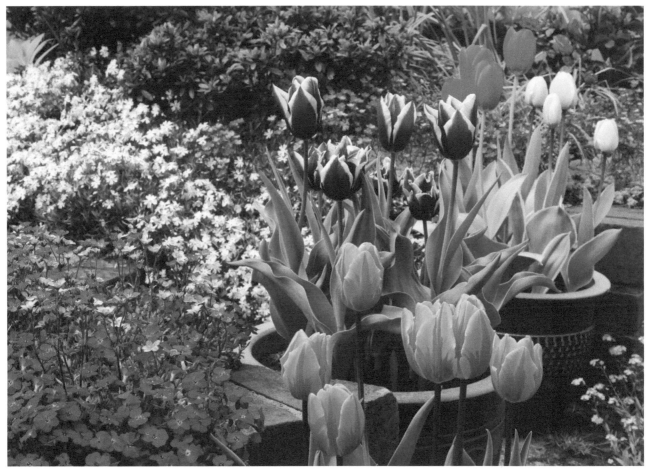

Colourful flowers in late spring border and patio pots filled with tulips.

Week 59
May 1ˢᵗ 2021

In UK, 34,216,087 have had 1ˢᵗ dose of vaccine and 14½ million two doses, all with expert know-how.
2/3 adult population given 1st dose of vaccine. Those aged 40+ can book appointments online now.

UK has ordered 60 million Pfizer booster shots. Rollout will begin in autumn for the most vulnerable.
Vaccine can cause sore arm, headache, fatigue, fever or sickness but lasts only 24 hours so tolerable.

4 in 10 councils have no Covid-19 deaths. 22m people live in areas that have no Covid deaths at all.
January, pandemic peak, 30,000 deaths but April down to 600. UK Covid deaths are 127,502 in total.

Public Health England study found one dose of vaccine reduces transmission by 38%-49% if infected.
Infections: England 1 in 1,010, Scotland 1 in 640, Wales 1 in 1,570, N. Ireland 1 in 940, ONS detected.

UK delivered vaccine to 11 of 14 British Overseas Territories, 250.000 doses arrived by sea and air.
Flew 8,000 miles to Falklands and 2,000 by sea to Tristan de Cunha, distance that's hard to compare.

In India, hospitals are being overwhelmed and many people are dying who could have been saved.
400,000 infections in 24hrs, 211,835 deaths total. One person is dying every 4 minutes, very grave.

UK sent 495 oxygen concentrators. They extract oxygen from air which will help some to breathe.
Also 120 non-invasive and 20 manual ventilators. 40 countries sent help which soon they'll receive.

Brazil has 2ⁿᵈ highest death toll in the world, 401,417. USA is first with 589,471 deaths from Covid.
Brazil criticizes President Bolsonaro for regarding coronavirus as a fantasy when the pandemic hit.

Turkey has entered lockdown for 3 weeks after surge of cases. Stay at home order proclaimed.
Opening up too soon in March, new variants, and Chinese Sinovac vaccine with 50% efficacy blamed.

Japan is in a 2-week lockdown just 2 months before Olympics. They could be behind closed doors.
A decision will be reached in June for Olympic start in July. Japan has already banned all visitors.

From Monday Australia will ban return of its citizens from India to prevent the Indian variant spread.
Those who fail to comply face up to 5 years in prison, A$66,000 fine, or both, authorities have said.

N. Ireland non-essential shops and gyms open, also self-contained accommodation and campsites.
15 from 3 households can meet in private gardens. Cafés, pubs and restaurants open but outside.

France starts lifting lockdown with schools May 3rd but 306 new deaths mean deaths remain high.
May 19th non-essential shops, theatres, outdoor cafés and restaurants open, rule of six will apply.

Government pilot scheme to see when UK can get back to gathering in large numbers has begun.
3,000 dance in nightclub in Liverpool with no face masks or social distancing but tests for everyone.

Residents in care home will no longer have to isolate for 2 weeks after going for a walk outside.
With a carer or designated visitor, they can visit relatives' gardens, public places and vote inside.

Campaign to raise £2.3m for memorial in St Paul's Cathedral starts for those who died of Covid-19.
Memorial for reflection of loved ones lost, open to all beliefs. A place that is tranquil and serene.

Week 60

May 8th 2021

Government has published the green list of countries that with tests can be visited from May 17th. France, Germany, Greece, Spain and USA are not included. The list will be reviewed in 3 weeks.

Green list includes Portugal, Gibraltar, Iceland, Israel, Singapore, New Zealand, Brunei, Australia, Falklands, Faroes, St Helena, Tristan de Cunha, Ascension Island, S. Sandwich Islands and S. Georgia.

PCR test 2 days after return and lateral flow before travel required. Turkey and Maldives on red list. Portugal includes Madeira and Azores but flight prices rise sharply, more bad news for the tourist.

UK ordered 60million Pfizer/BioNTech booster doses for possible start with vulnerable in September. Over 50m doses of vaccine delivered, 35m one dose and 17.7m two doses, lots more to go, however.

40+ offered vaccine in England, 45+ in Scotland, 40+ in Wales and 30+ N. Ireland. N.I is well ahead. Under 40s will be offered an alternative to AstraZeneca vaccine as a very rare blood clot risk with AZ.

Deaths continue to fall in UK. Friday, 15 deaths and 2,490 new infections with 81 deaths in a week. On January 20th, 1,820 deaths in 24 hrs and almost 60,000 new cases with 39,000 in hospital at peak.

Public Health England (PHE) elevated Indian virus variant subtype B.1617.2 to 'variant of concern'. More than 500 cases in Leicester, Bolton and London, 40 clusters, with cases in care homes we learn.

India continues to face rising surge of Covid cases. At present, responsible for 46% of cases globally. 18 year olds upwards eligible for vaccine but vaccines in short supply. 2% have been vaccinated only.

India had 400,000 cases and 4,000 deaths in a day, 23,000 deaths in 7 days. Such shocking numbers. Sputnik V vaccine has arrived from Russia. UK sent 1,000 more ventilators and 450 oxygen cylinders.

Government pledges 29.3m on top of 1.7m already promised to Porton Down to trace new variants. Labs will test 3000 blood samples a day for variants resistant to vaccines to help new developments.

76 days to Olympics but infections surge and restrictions continue. It may not go ahead as planned. Pfizer/BioNTech has offered jabs to all Olympic competitors and staff before they travel to Japan.

Germany starts to beat 3rd wave and fully vaccinated people can meet indoors without restrictions. China rewards its people with music festivals across the country as now they have few infections.

5,000 attended live music venue at Sefton Park, Liverpool, Sunday, part of government pilot scheme. Lateral flow test but no masks or social distancing. The Blossoms' pop music for many was a dream.

Also Sunday, World Snooker final at Crucible Theatre, Sheffield, filled 980 seats, 100% full capacity. 33% for first round of tournament, 50% second and 75% for semi-finals. All received with alacrity.

AZ vaccine loaded into boats, kept at -8C and for use within 24 hrs, has been taken up Amazon River. In remote communities, widespread vaccine hesitancy was met. 500 vaccines took 2 days to deliver.

'Gardeners beware of the frost' - May temperatures lower than normal with frosts on many a night. Significant damage to camellias and magnolias but the tulips have gone on and on so that's all right.

Week 61
May 15th 2021

Hugging is allowed from 17th May but advice is to avoid hugging face to face and to keep it short.
Vaccinated grandparents hugging grandchildren is low risk but who to hug needs some thought.

From Monday, six, or 2 households, can meet indoors and groups of 30 are able to meet outdoors.
Indoor visits and staying overnight is allowed. Care home residents allowed 5, not 2 visitors, 3 more.

Opening of restaurants and pubs for inside eating and drinking means we won't freeze or get wet.
But social distancing and service only at tables will reduce numbers and profits businesses will get.

Covid alert level reduced from level 4 to 3; virus circulating but transmission no longer rising or high.
Covid is a major pandemic globally. India and Nepal cases surge, Pakistan's Eid festival may amplify.

Monday in Scotland 6 people from 3 households can meet indoors and 8 from 8 households outside.
Pubs/restaurants open for food and drink inside. No social distancing and no rules on hugging abide.

Cinemas/ theatres open. Scotland moves level to 2, Glasgow and Moray stay 3 as many infections.
English travel traffic light system is adopted. Wales restaurants/pubs open indoors with restrictions.

PM anxious about spread of Indian virus variant; can't rule out restrictions or changes on June 21st.
Cases jumped from 520 to 1,313 in a week. 17 cases in Wales but in NW and London virus the worst.

Tricky finding B.1617.2 variant in testing. No data on infectivity or effect on vaccine efficacy as yet.
But Indian variant may be 50% more transmissible than Kent. Certainly, it continues to be a threat.

Surge testing in 15 areas. 100 nurses will go door to door in Bolton. Extra vaccine to Bolton supplied.
Increase is in the younger unvaccinated. Local feeling that offering vaccines to over 18s is justified.

Over 50s second dose will be accelerated from 12 to 8 weeks to increase immunity to new variants.
National average of infections 23 in 100,000, 193 in Bolton, 108 in Blackburn with Darwin residents.

38 and 39-year-olds can book jabs. All pregnant women and under 40s offered Pfizer or Moderna.
Vaccine has saved 11,700 from death, mostly 80+ year olds, and 33,000 entering hospital, a wonder.

Portugal is on the UK green travel list but 'State of Calamity' there has been extended to May 30th.
UK tourists welcome from Monday but negative PCR test in last 72 hours they have to arrive with.

4,000 attend Brit Awards at O2, no social distancing or masks as part of Government pilot scheme.
More than half audience are NHS Key workers, some having their first night out for a year, a dream.

60% of US have had at least one vaccination. FDA approved Pfizer for 12-15-year-olds, worthwhile.
Biden said fully vaccinated needn't wear masks inside or out. They can greet others with a smile.

Cities, states and businesses in US provide perks encouraging the having a vaccination decision.
Anything from free donuts, free beer, $50 gift voucher, $100 saving bond or chance to win a million.

Week 62

May 22nd 2021

Red means stop, green means go, but what does amber mean? To travellers it means 'great let's go'.
But to politicians it means only essential travel is all right, travel to amber countries a definite no-no.

Monday Heathrow was buzzing with travel to Portugal, also 150 flights to destinations on amber list.
France, Germany, Italy, Spain, US flights left. Travel to 170 amber countries 'legal', travellers insist.

EU discusses allowing fully vaccinated from non-EU. Spain lifts restrictions for UK arrivals 24th May.
Handy vaccine records are found on the NHS app and can be used as a vaccine passport for a stay.

Germany introduces ban on travel from UK except for residents and citizens who must quarantine.
UK quarantine spot-check team increased to 30,000. Fine of £10,000 for non-compliance is routine.

France has moved curfew back 2 hours to 9pm. Cinemas and museums open and cafés open outside.
Fully open June 9th. Non-essential shops open. From May 31st, vaccine for all adults they'll provide.

In England, 7 in 10 have had one jab and 4 in 10 are fully vaccinated. 37,250,365 first doses given.
Two jabs of Pfizer or AstraZeneca is 97% effective, data hospital medics and healthcare staff driven.

England extends vaccine eligibility to 32 & 33-year-olds, Wales 18+, N. Ireland 25+ and Scotland 30+.
Areas of Glasgow are offering 18-30-year-olds vaccine as Indian variant is making councils nervous.

Indian variant, B.1617.2, reported in 86 councils. Infections rose 30% from Monday to Wednesday.
Discovered in Hounslow, Hillingdon, Croydon, Bedford, Canterbury and Chelmsford to much dismay.

National Test and Trace provided no Indian arrivals data to eight NW councils 21st April to 11th May.
Technical hitch caused 700 cases not to be followed up, serious consequences from 3-week delay.

Increasing evidence vaccine protects from Indian variant but a strong hint it is highly transmissible.
Three-dose vaccine trial to monitor antibodies and immunity from variants started on those eligible.

Sewage testing for genetic fragments of virus is ramped up, now covers 2/3 of England's population.
500 sites test wastewater 4 times a week and new dedicated lab in Exeter tracks virus in circulation.

Infections continue to surge in India with 4,529 deaths on Wednesday creating a global daily record.
294,794 in total, US 602.656, Brazil 444,391, UK 127,710 and New Zealand 26 which we can applaud.

Scotland restricts travel to Bedford, Bolton and Blackburn with Darwen. Moray goes to level two.
Wales allows six from six different households indoors. Hugging isn't allowed but is under review.

Olympic committee confirms games will go ahead although 80% of the Japanese are very against it.
Only 5% of population vaccinated. Moderna and AZ only just joined Pfizer in the vaccines permitted.

May weather has been a real disappointment with unseasonably wet and windy weather this week.
Gales with storm force ten gusts battered the garden as lilac and azaleas were reaching their peak.

Turkey sounds attractive as a holiday destination but as it's on the amber list, it's out of our reach.
Lucky Cathedral Cheddar plastic wrappers reached Turkey. They even found their way onto a beach.

Week 63
May 29th 2021

Vaccination schedule has been very successful in UK. 45% of adults have had 2 doses, 75% just one.
30-year-olds eligible in England, 30+ in Scotland,18+ N. Ireland, Wales end of June. First round won.

Cases of Indian variant in UK have doubled in a week. ½ of infections in UK are now B.1.617.2 strain.
Hotspots Burnley, Bolton, Blackburn, Bedford, N. Tyneside, Hounslow, Kirklees and Leicester, again.

Government issued guidance on its website for hotspots which included severe travel restriction.
It backtracked as advice was seen as lockdown through stealth. For many, it brought total confusion.

Scotland extends level 3 for Glasgow for at least another week but is optimistic things will get better.
Rising cases are Indian variant-driven and businesses are finding it difficult to hold things together.

R number has risen, 1.0 – 1.1. On Friday, 4,182 new cases, 10 deaths and 916 in hospitals in England.
Bolton, 49 in hospital, 30-40s who've had only one jab, or no jab at all, but none had had a second.

PHE says one dose of Pfizer or AZ gives 50% immunity from Kent variant but only 33% from Indian.
But after 2 doses Pfizer 88% and AZ 66% from Indian. Important to get 2nd dose for extra protection.

European countries seeing spread in UK of Indian variant have their attention on avoidance focused.
Austria bans UK direct flights from June 1st and France introduces 7-day quarantine for UK May 31st.

No data indicates lockdown end June 21 in England could be delayed but decision may be changed.
Scientists suggest date for reopening should be postponed giving time for 2nd doses to be arranged.

Johnson & Johnson's Janssen one-dose vaccine, has just been approved in UK, available later in year.
EU authorizes use of Pfizer for 12 to 15-year-olds but no plan to vaccinate younger than 16 yet here.

Indian second wave has peaked in Delhi and other areas but in some regions, cases are still rising.
Cases peaked at 392,000 a day, now fallen to 200,000. 319,007 deaths which, sadly, isn't surprising.

Cummings launched stinging attack on PM and Matt Hancock in 7-hour testimony on Wednesday.
Cast doubt on PM's fitness for office, Matt Hancock's truthfulness and also pandemic enquiry delay.

New variant, C.36.3, first detected in Thailand amongst travellers from Egypt, has been found in UK.
109 cases identified and variant under investigation. We hope it won't prove yet another runaway.

Japan has extended its state of emergency another 3 weeks to end just a month before Olympics.
Argentina imposes new lockdown as cases soar. Vaccine rollout slow, say worst point in pandemic.

Findings from government mass event pilot scheme are positive. Only 15 in 58,000 got Covid-19.
Safely measures taken for FA cup, Liverpool club night, Brit Awards and no severe risk could be seen.

Sniffer dogs prove more accurate than lateral flow tests in detecting people who have Covid-19.
Could be used at airports and mass events so when trials are completed some good use is foreseen.

Fine weather is forecast at last. It's getting warmer and Sunday will be sunny and 20 degrees C.
Bank holiday Monday will be even warmer at 25C. Wonderful, now we're happy, rejoicing with glee.

JUNE 2021

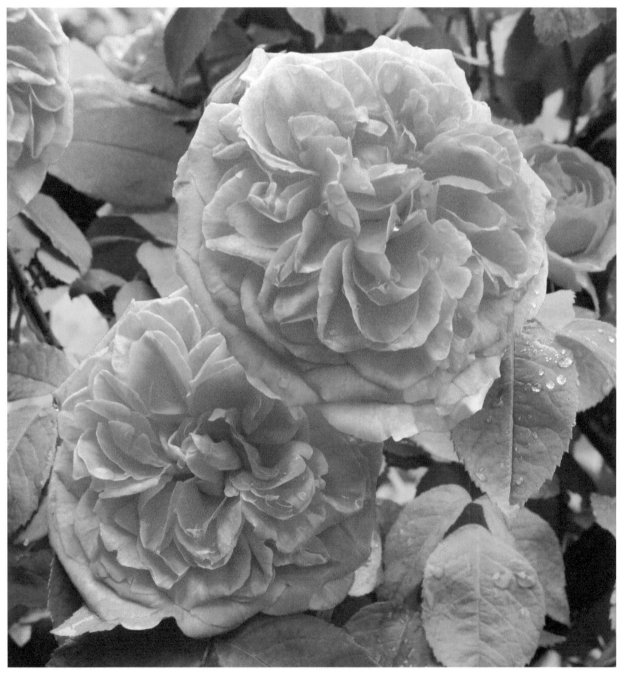

Fragrant Gertrude Jekyll roses after shower of rain.

Week 64
June 5th 2021

3rd June Portugal was removed from green travel list. Arrivals must quarantine after 4 am 8th of June.
Tourists change return flights, holidays cancelled and holiday industry angry at their sad misfortune.

Egypt, Sri Lanka, Afghanistan, Bahrain, Costa Rica, Sudan, Trinidad and Tobago all added to red list.
No countries added to green, so, for a staycation, book now; a chance to holiday is too good to miss.

WHO renames variants using Greek alphabet to avoid stigmatized labelling with country of origin.
Alpha/UK, Beta/S. African, Gamma/Brazilian, Delta/ Indian, Kappa/Australian. For many, foreign.

UK worried about variant from Nepal found in Portugal. WHO doesn't recognise it; they're sanguine.
It's Delta variant+K417N mutation found in Beta, highly infectious, may challenge efficacy of vaccine.

12,431 cases of Delta variant confirmed in UK up to June 2, up 79% on previous week. Is it 3rd wave?
Friday 6,238 cases,11 deaths, 954 in hospital. Hospitalization more likely with Delta variant, so grave.

Surge testing for Delta variant starts in Berkshire on Monday for 2 weeks. Everyone offered PCR test.
64 cases in 100,000 have been recorded when national average is only 18. Nipping it in bud is best.

MHRA have approved use of Pfizer/BioNTech for 12-15-year-olds in UK but no plans to vaccinate yet.
Blackburn with Darwen pleads for vaccine soon; secondary school infections are becoming a threat.

Vietnam reports surge of infections. Ho Chi Minh City starts mass testing with target 100,000 a day.
Virus is hybrid of Alpha and Delta strains. Cases doubled but good tracing system is now underway.

Peru updated Covid death toll from 69,342 to 180,764. It has world's highest death rate per capita.
It has registered 1.9m infections in a population of 33 million. Poor health care is clearly a big factor.

In UK, more than 75% of adults vaccinated with one dose and over 50% of adults given 2 injections.
39,758,428 have had first dose and 26, 422,302 second. A second assures much stronger protection.

In Wales, on Monday 3 households can meet indoors, 30 people outside. Alert level lowered to one.
Outdoor events, concerts, festivals, football matches possible, 4,000 standing, 10,000 sitting down.

Scotland's central region remains at level 2, Glasgow down from 3 to 2. Most of Scotland moves to 1.
8 from 3 households in café, 6 from 3 households in home, 12 from 12 families outside, so more fun.

Heathrow T3 now dedicated to direct flights from countries on red list, at last not mixing with green.
376,000 have reported long Covid for over a year, fatigue, muscle pain and a lot more in between.

Weather is iffy but okay as there's the Greek alphabet to learn moving our knowledge up a notch.
After delta comes epsilon, zeta, eta, theta and iota, later Sigma, a lens, and lastly, Omega, a watch.

Week 65
June 12th 2021

Vaccine for less wealthy countries is a major topic at G7 summit which started on Friday in Cornwall. UK, USA, Canada, France, Germany, Italy, Japan, plus EU representative discussed vaccine shortfall.

US pledged 500m vaccine doses, UK, Germany, France, Italy 100m doses and Japan 1 billion dollars. It's urgently needed for healthcare workers, vulnerable and to prevent further mutations of virus.

COVAX requires 11 billion doses for poorer countries but there is a problem with vaccine hesitancy. Population of poorer nations have many daily worries and don't see Covid-19 as an emergency.

Cases of Covid in Bolton are falling, help from army with vaccination and testing has been a success. Now Greater Manchester and Lancashire have cases surging. It's affecting 4 million people, no less.

Andy Burnham, G. Manchester mayor, asked for vaccine for 18+ to prevent spread; request denied. Advice is to meet outside, restrict travel in and out of area, work from home. Said to be only a guide.

25-29-year-olds became eligible for vaccination from Tuesday. It led to over a million appointments. Many people now have antibodies from vaccine or infections. 80% of all adults in UK it represents.

Saturday there were 7,738 cases, 1,089 hospitalisations and 12 deaths. Recently all three have risen. Deaths not high yet but the link between Covid-19 cases and deaths is only weakened not broken.

It has been found that Delta variant is 60% more transmissible than the highly transmissible Alpha. It's the dominant strain in UK. Now 90% of Covid cases are the variant first identified in India, Delta.

Delta cases doubled this week to 30,000. It's twice as likely to cause serious illness in the infected. Nearly 2/3 of Delta cases not vaccinated and more than half of those who died totally unprotected.

Pfizer is updating its vaccine with variant sequencing for use against new strains which may emerge. Oxford starts trials with vaccine booster which produces strong neutralising antibodies against surge.

This week there's been endless speculations as to what will happen on 'Freedom Day', June 21st. Brides with more than 30 guests invited debate how to uninvite guests if worst comes to worst.

PM says it will be a cautious but irreversible lifting of restrictions but is not committing on 21st June. Said data was being examined and he'd let us all know on Monday 14th. Fortunately that's very soon.

Dating apps ask users to include their vaccine status. They hope to encourage jabs for those single.
They're giving benefits, virtual badges and stickers announcing 'Jabbed, single and ready to mingle'.

Pop-up campsites in farms, pubs and stately homes are legal for 56 days, too short for staycations.
Group, 'Carry on Camping', is campaigning for a 6-month extension to pop-up campsite regulations.

G7 had Cornish 'mizzle', mist and drizzle, but Biden's praise for the countryside was unaffected.
Friday it was Eden Centre dinner with Royals. Weather is irrelevant there so experience perfected.

Week 66

June 19th 2021

Monday 14th June, PM gave us the news we were expecting. All restrictions won't be lifted 21st June. For hospitality, nightclubs, shows, concerts and mass events this means disaster, not just misfortune.

Restriction on numbers for weddings and wakes is lifted but social distancing must still be observed. No one can dance at weddings, but in 2 weeks, restrictions reviewed. On the outcome PM reserved.

PM 'confident' no delay will be needed beyond 19th July. More people will have had 2 jabs by then. In Scotland level 0 delayed 3 weeks by Delta variant. Welsh delay lifting restrictions for same reason.

Delta variant is dominant in Wales with 488 cases. Mark Drakeford said they are in the third wave. Chief Scientific Adviser says 'virus will be with us forever'. Must accept this if lives are to be saved.

On Monday 800 people admitted to hospital, twice the number admitted on Monday previous week. Most had 1 jab or no jab, but 1 in 20 fully vaccinated for over 2 weeks and that's not news we seek.

One dose has been found to reduced hospitalisation and serious illness by 75% and 2 doses by 90%. Friday there were 10,476 new cases, 1,252 hospitalisations and 11 deaths, all rising to some extent.

Only 40% of people who test positive after being fully vaccinated show symptoms of coronavirus. They are less likely to have a high level of virus in their system than unvaccinated or be infectious.

Surge testing for Delta variant is being carried out across England and Scotland to try to curb spread. ONS says 1 in 540 people are infected but 1 in 2,480 in East and 1 in 180 in NW as NW is way ahead.

React-1 study shows spread driven by the young, 5-12-year-olds and 18-24s who are unvaccinated. Pfizer is authorized for 12-18-year-olds in UK but reasons for use on children at present attenuated.

Tuesday, 23/24-year-olds invited to book jabs and on Friday, over 18s. Over 42m have had first dose. Symptoms for Delta variant different from previous variants; sore throat, headache and runny nose.

Cruise companies have cancelled many holidays as had catered for non-social distancing on cruises. Monday, 5-day quarantine in Italy for UK. The precaution against spread of Delta variant it chooses.

Government confirms vaccination compulsory for carers in care homes, 1/3 at present unvaccinated. Employees given 16 weeks to get vaccinated or lose their job. Employers with vacancies are agitated.

8-month-long 11pm curfew ends in France and masks not needed outdoors, except when queueing. In Germany, fully vaccinated people can do more. In Italy, indoor service allowed, curfew is lifting.

Dogs can identify compounds produced during Covid infection which could be useful at mass events. May be possible to create device which can identify odour. This would be tremendous advancement.

Week 67

June 26th 2021

16 travel destinations were added to UK green list but Malta is the only one not on a watch list.
You can travel to the others but should they turn amber, it'll be quarantining at home for the tourist.

The 15 on green watch are Caymans, Dominica, Madeira, Bermuda, Antigua, Anguilla, Antarctica,
Turks and Caicos, Barbados, Balearics, Virgin Islands, Pitcairn Islands, Montserrat and Grenada.

Plans are afoot to drop quarantine for the fully vaccinated returning from countries on amber list.
It'll happen 'later in summer' said transport Secretary Grant Shapps. Delay will allow more fairness.

83% of adults have had one dose but only 61% have had two; need chance to even up percentages.
18+ booked 6 jab slots every second online. They're keen for freedom with closer acquaintances.

Pop-up vaccine centres in stadiums, football grounds and shopping centres attracted long queues.
One day, 221,534 1st doses given and 177,813 second. The 'Grab a Jab' success for adults continues.

Over 50s in minority ethnic groups in parts of London are refusing jabs, vaccination progress is slow.
Hackney 17,000 refuse jabs. Double-decker bus used as mobile centre in areas where take-up is low.

Scotland's infections are high; won't move to level 0 till 19th July, but all restrictions to lift 9th August.
The goal is to have all adults fully vaccinated by 12th September. On this date, they're totally focused.

UK has gone from having the lowest number of infections in Europe to the country with the highest.
Angela Merkel warns Europe it's 'on thin ice'. Delta variant will cause 90% of infections by August.

Friday, UK 15,810 new cases, 1,485 in hospital and 18 deaths. Infections rose by 5,000 Wednesday.
R rate is 1.2-1.4, infection is spreading. 10 infected will infect 12 to 14. Delta variant now a runaway.

There was a 46% increase in infections last week. 60% of cases unvaccinated but 20% fully jabbed.
Biggest increase is in group aged 17-24, most likely to mix. 2 doses of vaccine they won't have had.

Infections amongst younger people and even hospitalisation results in recovery that is usually ace.
Trial starts where fully vaccinated test each day instead of isolating after contacting a positive case.

React study finds at least 2 m people who developed Covid symptoms went on to have long Covid.
Tiredness, shortness of breath, headaches or chest pains Covid induced creates continual invalids.

Seven vaccines are being tested to find the most effective booster. Results end of August not sooner.
Vaccines to be used as third dose are Pfizer, AstraZeneca, Valneva, Janssen, Novavax and Moderna.

Stadiums at Japanese Olympics will be filled to 50% capacity with a maximum of 10,000 spectators.
Masks, no cheering and having to go straight home afterwards mandatory and all rather vexatious.

People are buying large inflatable pools complete with slides, some 15 feet, for staycations at home.
Bobbing around on a lilo in garden puts a strain on water supply and makes for expensive outcome.

July 1st Guernsey will open borders to UK tourists who are lucky enough to be doubly vaccinated.
Weekly rhyming reports will end as I'm off to Guernsey. I'll return when I'm fully regenerated.

JULY 2021

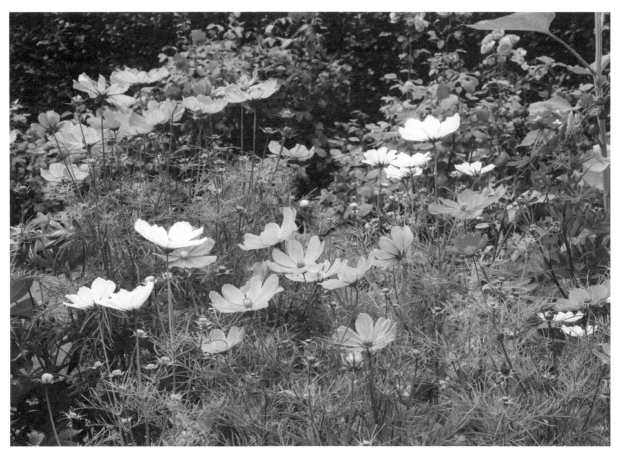

Pink and white cosmos flowers in summer border.

Week 71

July 20th 2021

'Freedom Day' Monday, July 19th. Masks no longer mandatory, no social distancing, nightclubs open. Restrictions have been lifted but Covid cases rise. The link with vaccine is weakened but not broken.

The world looks on, some in horror, as England starts what is regarded by many as an experiment. PM explains 'If we don't open up now, when can we?' Waiting until winter would seem improvident.

16th July positive cases in Scotland were 1 in 90, in England 1 in 95, NI 1 in 290 and Wales 1 in 360. Hospitalisations are doubling every 3 weeks in England warns Chief Scientific Adviser Chris Whitty.

Vaccination reduces serious illness and death. PHE found AZ 60% effective against Delta, 88% Pfizer. 87.8% of adults have had 1st dose and 68.3% 2nd. Adults to be offered 2 doses by end of September.

Health Secretary has Covid, PM and Chancellor self-isolating. Cases are now higher than in January. June 29th 20,479 new cases, July 17th 54,674, 96 deaths and 4,567 in hospital today. Rise looks scary.

Over 1 m children are off school for Covid-related reasons, 47,200 with confirmed cases of virus. School year is finishing. PM thinks if restrictions are lifted now the decision will be less contentious.

Young queued for nightclubs to open at midnight 18th July and they bopped until 4 the next morning. Full vaccination may be mandatory in nightclubs end of September. Club owners object to warning.

'Ping Pandemic' is in the news. 618,903 people 'pinged' in a week threatening essential services. Bosses can apply for exemption on an individual basis for critical workers in the right circumstances.

19th July - Scotland moved to level 0. FM will lift all restrictions August 9th. Masks remain mandatory. Wales lifts number restriction outside. Restrictions to be lifted August 7th. Masks mostly obligatory.

Sainsbury's, M & S, Lidl, Tesco, Morrison's, Aldi and Asda all urge customers to wear masks in stores. London Mayor, Sadiq Khan, makes masks compulsory on London transport. For safety 'rule' endures.

Fully vaccinated can travel to amber countries, except for France, without quarantining on return. PCR test 3 days before travel home and 2nd day after return, costs £50-£100. It will re-entry govern.

Delta variant and Beta variant fuel France's 4th wave as infections surge. 'Health passes' introduced. Passes needed for cinemas, museums and theme parks. Restaurants, transport and malls proposed.

15 research studies started into symptoms and possible treatments for long Covid-19 after virus. £20M funding from National Institute for Health Research. Brain fog and lung damage will be focus.

JCVI advice is that children 12-16 vulnerable to serious illness from Covid-19 can have Pfizer vaccine. Pfizer for 12-17-year-olds in households where an adult is immunosuppressed is also to be routine.

Holiday bookings surged 5th July when PM announced restrictions to end 19th. EasyJet sales up 400%. Campsites, B&B, hotels and self-catering staycations sell out to meet a need for a holiday well spent.

After weeks of wet weather, the sun came out and temperatures soared hitting 31.6C on 18th July. Beaches were packed and sun cream needed as UK celebrated in a heatwave with a clear blue sky.

AUGUST 2021

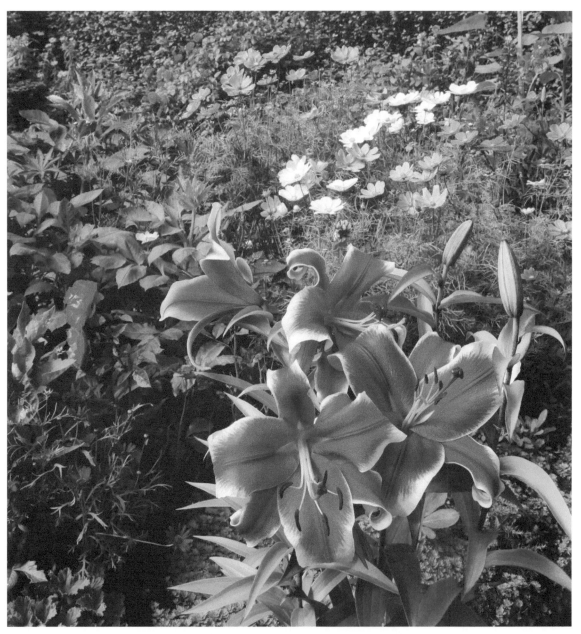

Stargazer lilies and cosmos flowers.

Week 73
August 11ᵗʰ 2021

It was announced on 10ᵗʰ August that more than 75% of UK adults are now fully vaccinated.
4ᵗʰ August JCVI approved Pfizer for 16 and 17-year-olds but only 1 dose at present advocated.

Vaccines are working well but cases, hospitalisations and deaths still remain quite considerable.
10ᵗʰ August deaths peaked at 146, cases lowered, 23,510, hospitalisation under 6,000 and stable.

Vaccination among 18-25-year-olds is low. Discount taxi rides and take-away incentives offered.
Sussex University offers a jackpot draw. 5 prizes of £5,000 for those doubly vaccinated proffered.

Wales and Scotland lifted restrictions 7ᵗʰ and 9ᵗʰ August but masks in indoor spaces they'll retain.
Mandatory mask-wearing in shops, medical centre settings and on public transport will remain.

Isolation after contact with Covid for fully vaccinated no longer required in Scotland and Wales,
Although Scotland does require a PCR test after contact. England's wait until 16ᵗʰ August prevails.

Green, amber and red travel lists were updated August 5ᵗʰ. Mexico joins red list causing major upset.
Germany, Austria, Norway, Latvia, Romania, Slovenia, Slovakia turn green. Travel there our best bet.

France is no longer 'Amber Plus' so the doubly vaccinated can return without having to quarantine.
India, Bahrain, Qatar and UAE move from red to amber so returning from these is now just routine.

Fully vaccinated travellers arriving from the EU and US no longer are required to isolate for 10 days;
Norway and Switzerland included. Spain was almost put on red list but just missed it in this phase.

Plans for booster shots with flu jabs for vulnerable are going ahead and will start in September.
Prof Pollard, vaccine team leader, says supplies sent to countries short of vaccine would be better.

Nine million doses of the AstraZeneca vaccine are on their way from UK to COVAX for distribution.
Parts of Africa where only 1% of people have been vaccinated will be happy with this contribution.

Scientists in Sweden are developing vaccine in powder form which is inhaled and tolerates over 40C.
Perfect for vaccinating in hot, less developed countries as it would make delivery simpler and easy.

Pfizer and Moderna passed as safe for pregnant women. Best interval between jabs under review.
US have made Covid-19 vaccination mandatory for the military and for all the federal workers too.

In Italy, travellers will need green Covid pass to board plane. For public venues, it is also obligatory. France introduces Covid-19 health pass which is compulsory for access to venues with more than 50.

International cruises recommenced on August 2nd. Virgin cruises have overhauled liners for safety. Air purifiers were fitted and ventilation increased. All passengers and crew must be vaccinated fully.

Prof Dame Sarah Gilbert who designed the Oxford/AZ vaccine was honoured in Queen's birthday list. AZ doses have been sent to 170 countries. There's now a Barbie Doll in Sarah's image; a nice twist.

OCTOBER 2021

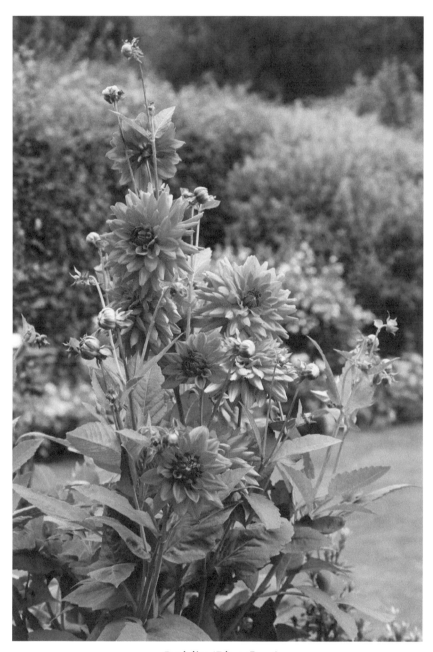

Dahlia 'Blue Boy'

Week 84
October 21ˢᵗ 2021

Legal restrictions ended in England on July 19ᵗʰ but now Covid cases are rising again. All is not well. Tuesday there were 223 deaths and today 115 deaths, 52,009 new cases with 8,142 in hospital.

Children account for many infections. 12 to 17-year-olds' single-dose vaccine must be given faster. Immunity wanes after 6 months and over 50s are being encouraged to take up booster jab offer.

New antiviral drugs await approval, Molnupiravir by Merck, Sharp & Dohme and Ritonavir by Pfizer. Health Minister, Sajid Javid, says there's no need for more restrictions; others appear wiser.

Scotland, Wales, N. Ireland masks are mandatory on public transport and in many venues. Covid passports essential for nightclub entry and mass events confirms their different views.

Green and amber travel lists have been scrapped. Fully vaccinated only need 2-day PCR test. Others need PCR departure, 2-day and 8-day return tests with a 10-day self-isolation behest.

October 24ᵗʰ lateral flow tests will replace PCR tests giving travel a cheaper and easier twist. Panama, Columbia, Venezuela, Peru, Ecuador, Haiti, Dominican Republic are on the red list.

Novavax vaccine has not been submitted for approval; doubly vaccinated in trial are upset. They're being given 2 Pfizer jabs. Novavax is 90% effective but travel rules have to be met.

UK cancelled 100M doses of French Valneva vaccine as believed it wouldn't gain approval. It uses inactivated Sars-CoV-2, can be stored in fridge; it's as effective as AZ so beneficial.

Mutation AY.4.2 or 'Delta Plus', has been identified, scientists are not sure what this means. Responsible for 6% UK cases, it's 10-15% more transmissible and could undermine vaccines.

B1.621, 'Mu' variant, Mu=12th, was identified as a variant of interest by WHO 30ᵗʰ August. Found in 39 countries, mostly US and thought to threaten vaccines but Delta rules as robust.

751,978 US Covid deaths make pandemic deadliest in US history. 675,000 flu deaths in 1918. At start 242m cases worldwide and 4.92m deaths from coronavirus were totally unforeseen.

6.5B doses of vaccine have been administered in 196 countries but distribution is not ideal. China 154.3 doses per 100 people, France 143.5, UK 138.9, India 70 but Africa, in areas, nil.

Over ¾ of vaccine doses produced have been used in just 10 countries said the WHO envoy.
Plane bearing AstraZeneca doses finally arrived in Antarctica to the research station's joy.

Over 50s can dial 119 for booster shot if it's 1 week past 6 months since their second jab.
Excellent news and as booster jabs 96% more effective than two jabs, this news is truly fab.

NOVEMBER 2021

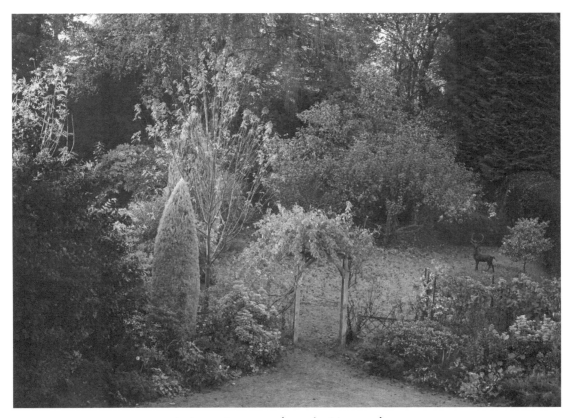

Late autumn colour in November

Week 88
November 20th 2021

'Storm clouds are gathering' over Europe. 15th November, Boris warned of a new wave of infections.
Full lockdown starts in Austria next week. They're unable to leave home with just a few exceptions.

Angela Merkel said the 4th wave was sweeping Germany. 65,000 infections recorded on Thursday.
67% of population vaccinated, 18+ offered booster jabs, unvaccinated need jabs fast without delay.

In the Netherlands, 80% of over 18s have had both jabs but infections are still surging relentlessly.
They've introduced a limited lockdown. Bars and restaurants required to close at 8 pm; very early.

Austria is taking the threat a step further. Vaccination will be made mandatory from next February.
Infections in Spain and France are increasing. They're taking measures but at present just cautionary.

England with high but stable infections has all its eggs in the vaccine basket. May be rather risky.
Thursday 46,807 new cases, 8,174 hospitalised, 199 deaths. Many 5–9-year-olds infected is a worry.

15 m have had booster jabs in England but residents of remote places struggle to get their shots.
Elderly asked to drive 50 miles for a jab, returning in the dark, are unhappy about their vaccine slots.

25% of 12-15-year-olds have been given a single jab and 16 & 17-year-olds are eligible for a 2nd jab.
Over 40s qualify for booster jab six months after being fully vaccinated. Progress is certainly not bad.

World Health Organization (WHO) is 'very worried' about spread of Covid-19 infections in Europe.
Calls for more mask-wearing and faster delivery of the Covid vaccine to help stem the virus' gallop.

US have authorised Pfizer vaccine for 5–11-year-olds and over 18s are being offered booster shots.
India has delivered a billion doses of vaccine. 70% have had one dose and that is reducing hot spots.

Some people failed to develop Covid after having close contact with people infected and contagious.
They were found to have Covid-fighting T-cells, possibly produced by the common cold coronavirus.

In Wales, Covid passes needed from Monday 15 November for cinemas, theatres and concert halls.
In N. Ireland, Covid passports necessary for pubs, restaurants, night clubs and any mass venues at all.

April 2022 vaccination will be mandatory for all front-line NHS staff providing close patient contact.
11th November full vaccination became mandatory for care home staff. It ended many a contract.

Anti-viral pill Molnupiravir has been approved in UK. Can be given twice daily to a vulnerable patient. May be taken at home. It must be given within 5 days of infection if it's to be an effective treatment.

Vax has been declared the 2021 word of the year by the Oxford English Dictionary, so we're told. With double-vaxxed, anti-vaxxer, unvaxxed and getting vaxxed, multiple uses for the word unfold.

At last, doubly vaccinated can fly to Australia and meet up with family they haven't seen for years. US opened borders to fully vaxxed in 33 countries, including UK. Travellers will shed joyous tears.

It's been unseasonably warm of late. Trees still have leaves and plants are flowering in the garden. Next week sees change. Temperatures will drop and snow fall. We'll need a pullover or a cardigan.

DECEMBER 2021

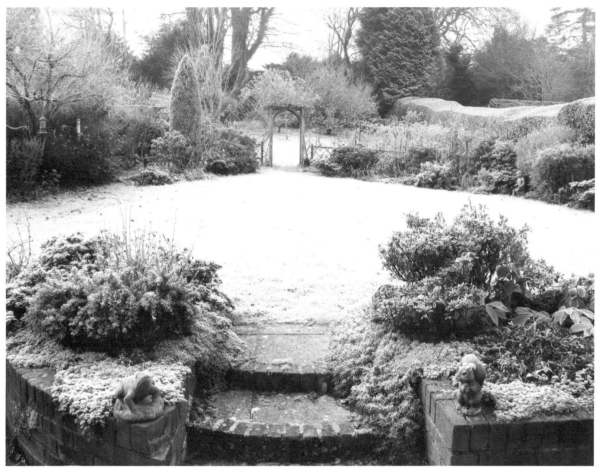

Frosty December garden

Week 90
December 4th 2021

Omicron variant was first identified in South Africa and reported to WHO on 24th November 2021. Omicron is 15th letter in Greek alphabet. 'O' is pronounced 'oh' but in general use, it's 'o' as in on.

The Omicron variant became a 'variant of concern' as it has many mutations and may avoid vaccines. B 1.1529 is spreading fast in South Africa. The world needs urgently to work out what this means.

32 mutations have been found on Omicron spike protein, 10 on 'receptor-binding domain' (RBD). RBD is key part of virus allowing it to gain entry into cells. Infection spread is bound to be speedy.

Midday 26th November, UK put 6 African countries on 'red travel list' and all flights were cancelled. Non-UK residents are banned from UK. Government is aware the situation must not be mishandled.

26th November, 59 cases were confirmed in South Africa, Israel, Belgium, Hong Kong and Botswana. 2 cases identified in UK next day, both S. African arrivals. Sajid Javid said, 'Pandemic is far from over'.

PM announced that on 30th November, masks would be mandatory in shops and on public transport. Masks already mandatory on transport and in shops Scotland, Wales & N. Ireland with forethought.

2-day tests for 'arrivals' to move from LFTs to PCRS. Isolation will be essential until a negative result. Contacts with Omicron infection must isolate 10 days, even fully vaccinated; for workers it's difficult.

Evidence is emerging that Omicron can evade the vaccine. One infection in Israel evaded a booster. Threat Omicron presents won't be known for weeks, a 'highly uncertain' size of wave for the future.

Moderna is testing its vaccines against Omicron and looking at 2 candidates suitable for a booster. Study found best protection from the Omicron variant was given by boosters of Moderna or Pfizer.

News 2nd December, Pfizer is working on booster to combat Omicron. It could be ready in 100 days. Pfizer has supplied 3 billion doses of vaccine and will produce 4 billion next year. It gains our praise.

UK has ordered 60m doses of Moderna and 54m of Pfizer. They will be delivered over next 2 years. Deal includes access to modified vaccine to combat Omicron, if needed, and emerging variant fears.

Pfizer is to produce a new formulation of their vaccine. It can be kept for 3 months in a refrigerator. In parts of Africa, less than 1 in 20 are vaccinated. This new vaccine could help vaccination go faster.

Germany is to ban unvaccinated people from some sectors, non-essential shops and leisure facilities.
Dec. 1st UK government issued advice to take lateral flow tests, not to cancel our Christmas parties.

UK has approved a new monoclonal antibody treatment, Sotrovimab, which reduces severe illness.
Sotrovimab binds to virus to stop it entering cells. Delivered as drip, it could reduce impact of virus.

30 Nov - 39,716 Covid cases, 7,631 in hospital, 141 deaths. Deaths from Delta variant are still high.
5.2m people have died globally. Total deaths in UK 144,285, US 782,000. A waste you can't justify.

The garden looks sad too now it's winter. It's drab with no flowers, fallen leaves and bare trees.
Pots full of bulbs show no sign of life, but they offer promise. It's best to lie low rather than freeze.

A Covid Cautious Cruise

Airports aren't attractive, the pandemic has seen to that.
But what about cruises, they're easier. Isn't that a fact?

But still, the chance of catching Covid is lurking everywhere.
In the taxi, you must wear a mask just to get you there.

You're required to be fully vaccinated, that's the only stipulation.
So, show your NHS QR code and you'll end their speculation.

The lateral flow test queue is long, slow-moving and outside.
There's a biting December wind and just nowhere you can hide.

Once on the ship and in your cabin, then get on and unpack.
As everything is done for you, you'll quickly get the knack.

Your holiday has started; relax, it will all work out fine.
But remember to wear a mask outside your cabin all the time.

You can take it off to eat and drink, it wouldn't work if you couldn't.
But if you want to leave the table without a mask, you really shouldn't.

Hand sanitiser dispensers you'll find all dotted around the ship.
So, give it a squirt when you're passing by and use it throughout the trip.

Each morning on your way to breakfast, your path you'll find is intercepted.
A temperature gun aimed at your head. It's routine so just accept it.

For a visit to some countries, you may find a PCR test has to be arranged.
A time slot for your test you're given and for a negative certificate exchanged.

But should your test be positive, be warned and bear in mind,
You'll stay onshore in a red hotel and simply be left behind.

When you arrive back home again, a wonderful holiday enjoyed,
You'll find you need another PCR but you shouldn't be annoyed.

You've been well fed and kept so safe; the crew have seen to that.
The only downside maybe is you've over-eaten and now you're far too fat.

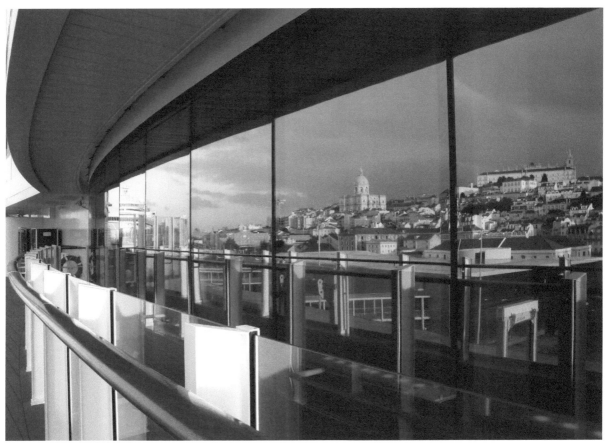

Lisbon reflected in cruise ship window.

Omicron s-gene Dropout.

The presence of the Covid-19 virus in a sample during a PCR test is detected by the presence of 3 genes. If one of these genes, the s-gene, is missing, the variant can almost certainly be classified as Omicron. S-gene dropout means the s-gene is not present. The Omicron variant has dangerous mutations of the spike protein which the virus uses to enter cells. This means this variant has the ability to penetrate cells more easily. It is not uncommon for those who have received a Pfizer booster jab to become infected with the Omicron variant. A booster jab is thought to give around 88% protection from severe illness.

Week 91

December 11ᵗʰ 2021

On Sunday 5ᵗʰ December, Omicron cases were rising. Transmission in the community had begun. Cases increased to 246 from 160 on Sunday and by Monday, there were 336 cases of Omicron.

Covid may cause a 4ᵗʰ wave and could put more people in hospital but there is massive uncertainty. Already 30% of cases in London are Omicron but it's impossible at this stage to know for certainty.

US study showed vaccine boosters offer some protection. Best results given by Pfizer and Moderna. Pfizer says booster will give 75% protection from Omicron, as much as two jabs gave us from Delta.

Nigeria added to the 'red list' 6ᵗʰ of December. Greece introduces compulsory vaccine for over 60s. Omicron found in 17 US states and 57 countries. It's 4 times more transmissible than Delta, a crisis.

R number is rising, 7ᵗʰ December England 0.9–1.1, Scotland 0.8-1.1, Wales 0.8-1, and N. Ireland 0.9-1. Infections in S. Africa increased x4 in a few days, rose from 4,000 to 16,000 with statistics on the run.

7ᵗʰ December mandatory LFT tests 48 hours before leaving for home became 'PCRs pre-departure'. Those abroad when change came in had to buy PCR tests in order to fill in the passenger locator.

PM announced move to Plan B on 8ᵗʰ December with 568 confirmed cases of Omicron in the UK. Face masks will be compulsory in most indoor venues, other than hospitality. Omicron is a runaway.

Work from home guidance announced by PM. It's part of Plan B and on 10ᵗʰ December it'll start. PM said, 'Go to work if you must but work from home if you can'. We must all try not to lose heart.

NHS Covid Pass will be mandatory in specific settings. It uses proof of negative test or vaccination. Nightclubs will only accept entry with NHS Covid Pass. 15ᵗʰ December that will come into operation.

Friday 10th December, new cases peaked at 59, 610, there were 120 deaths and 7,423 in hospital. Those with weakened immune system offered a 3ʳᵈ jab, plus booster 3 months later, as vulnerable.

Saturday 11ᵗʰ December, Omicron cases rose to 1,898. Symptoms found to differ from Delta variant. Extreme fatigue, scratchy throat, runny nose, headache and body pains primary symptoms present.

Omicron variant is classified as s-gene dropout. Not all labs can differentiate it from other variants. 3 genes indicate virus present in sample. Omicron has s-gene missing, 2 only in specimen fragments.

In Scotland, all contacts of Omicron must isolate for 10 days even if testing negative and vaccinated. Omicron variant doubling every 2.5 –3 days. This means Delta will soon be by Omicron dominated.

In care homes, only 3 visitors allowed plus one essential care worker. An attempt to reduce spread. With so much uncertainty, we don't know where we stand and many at their wit's end with Covid.

A cruise liner in December 3 times failed to dock in strong winds. Ship forced to continue to roam. A passenger explained, 'It's the pandemic that's responsible. The captain is working from home'.

Week 92

December 18ᵗʰ 2021

PM Boris Johnson announced: a 'tidal wave of Omicron is coming', 'get boosted', you mustn't delay.
Nicola Sturgeon: 'the tsunami is about to hit', Mark Drakeford 'Storm of Omicron is coming our way'.

Chris Whitty said, 'The peak will come fast but recede just as quickly'. Sadly, it's sure to be damaging.
Delta and Omicron are both causing infections. Delta's stable but Omicron's increase is staggering.

New cases climb each day. Wednesday 78,610, Thursday 88,376, Friday 93,045. They keep on rising.
Hospitalisations are becoming elevated. Deaths more or less stable. We must try to keep sanguine.

R number is between 3 and 5, 1 person with Covid is infecting 3 to 5 people, making numbers grow.
Omicron variant is doubling in less than 2 days and figures are much higher than test results show.

France has banned UK tourists and work trip visits, although France itself has 50,000 cases a day.
Countries with test and vaccination restrictions are Portugal, Spain, US, India, Hong Kong & Norway.

Our Queen has cancelled pre-Christmas dinner at Windsor with three generations of close family.
She felt it would put people's festive arrangements at risk, a decision that couldn't have been easy.

Midweek, Omicron variant became dominant in England and Scotland by 53% and 51% respectively.
Masks and home working stopped Omicron doubling every 2 days. It's starting to work effectively.

Booster jab may provide 88% protection from severe illness. Goal is to administer 1m jabs each day.
Thursday 3/4m booster jabs administered and Friday 861,302. We're hoping they'll be our mainstay.

12 Dec - Covid alert level rose to Level 4, transmission high and the NHS increasingly under pressure.
Hospitalisations could soar and may reach 3,000 a day, causing care to become difficult to deliver.

Dec 13 over 30s asked to book booster shots. Dec 15 18+ invited if second jab at least 3 months ago.
Anyone over 18 encouraged to either make an appointment or attend a walk-in centre and just go.

3000 centres have opened up across England with theatres and sports halls being brought into use.
Pregnant women are prioritised at tailored vaccine sites where they won't have to wait in queues.

Dec 14 vaccinated people must take lateral flow tests daily if in contact with anyone testing positive.
But 'NHS online' has run out of lateral flow tests. Demand at the moment is particularly intensive.

20,000 vaccinator volunteers signed up. Boris said Omicron variant must be given 'both barrels'.
750 armed forces personnel brought in to give jabs. The formation of the new 'jabs army' unravels.

Chris Whitty said in 5 years, polyvalent vaccines will protect us from 'New variants as they come in'.
In next 2-3 years new variants will lead to revaccination or booster shots as far as we can determine.

18 Dec - Sadiq Kahn declared major incident in London; emergency services are failing to keep pace.
4 out of 5 cases in London are Omicron, 10,000 more cases today. Are we starting to lose the race?

US zoos are vaccinating the animals. Those that are in close contact with people, especially big cats.
Animals chosen are primates, lions, tigers and jaguars, as well as the amazing Egyptian fruit bats.

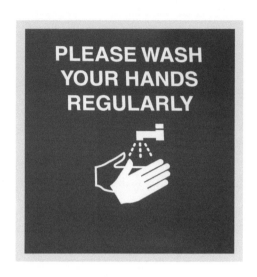

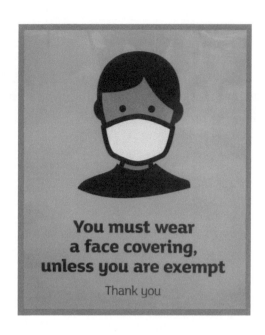

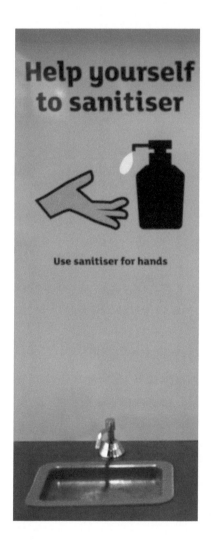

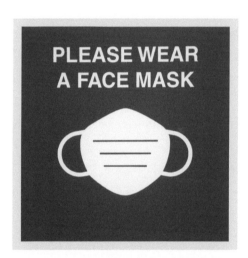

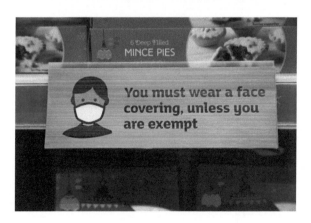

Signs popped up again everywhere when the Omicron variant spread like wildfire.

Week 93
December 25th 2021

It's Christmas Day and there's a feeling of optimism in the air. We hope all is as good as it seems.
With no restrictions, we can entertain as we please and have the family Christmas of our dreams.

News that the Omicron variant is less severe than Delta puts icing on the Christmas cake as well.
Analysis of results based on Omicron are 'promising' said Sajid Javid, but it's 'still too early to tell'.

Data from South Africa, Denmark, Scotland and England indicates it's likely to be 40-75% less potent.
Imperial College says 40-45%, Scotland 65%, S. Africa 75%, UK Health Security Agency 50-70 percent.

Many have Covid at present. 1 in 35 in England, 1 in 65 Scotland and 1 in 45 Wales sick last week.
In London, it was 1 in 20. ONS estimated 1.7m infected in UK and spread still hasn't reached its peak.

New cases grew as the week progressed 106,122 Wednesday, 119,789 Thursday and 122,186 Friday.
It's thought about half suffering from a cold actually have Covid; symptoms are very similar they say.

Quarantine for the vaccinated, after negative results days 6 and 7, has now been reduced to 7 days.
Many join family who would have been isolating over Christmas and a glass of bubbly they can raise.

Hospitalisations: Wednesday 8,008, Thursday 8,216, Friday 8,240; numbers rising, no sign of ease.
Sheer number of infections is responsible for admissions; it's not Omicron causing severe disease.

26 December in Scotland, Wales and N. Ireland nightclubs are to close and other restrictions applied.
Limit 100 standing, 200 sitting indoors and 500 outside in Scotland. Mass Hogmanay events denied.

Wales and N. Ireland introduce rule of 6 in pubs and restaurants with table service only, masks worn.
Wales 2-metre rule in shops, limit on outdoor events 50, 30 indoors, freedom is to be withdrawn.

Denmark is in 3rd wave. Theatres, cinemas and amusement parks close. Most now work from home.
Netherlands starts month of lockdown. 4 visitors allowed over Christmas so no one should be alone.

Xi'an in China is in lockdown. Travel to Germany from France, Denmark, Norway and UK is restricted.
Masks are now mandatory outdoors in Spain and Italy. Israel over 60s are to be 4 times vaccinated.

UKHSA say booster jabs wane against Omicron after 10 weeks. Immunity from Omicron falls quickly.
Infections will cause symptoms but admission to hospital and severe disease is 50 to 70% less likely.

Monoclonal antibody drug Sotrovimab is 79% effective if given to vulnerable people in first few days.
It's administered through a drip in outpatients; cancer and transplant patients will be eligible always.

22 Dec – FDA authorised use of Paxlovid, antiviral drug, produced by Pfizer in prescription pill form.
It should be given within 5 days of symptoms appearing. Can be prescribed and then taken at home.

PM says getting vaccinated will act as an 'invisible and invaluable present' for others this Christmas.
Some vaccination centres in England stay open. They'll give a gift that to some could prove priceless.

This Christmas people are asked to do lateral flow tests before mixing with others at holiday fests.
Children are on board. Many letters to Santa this Christmas include a luxury box of lateral flow tests.

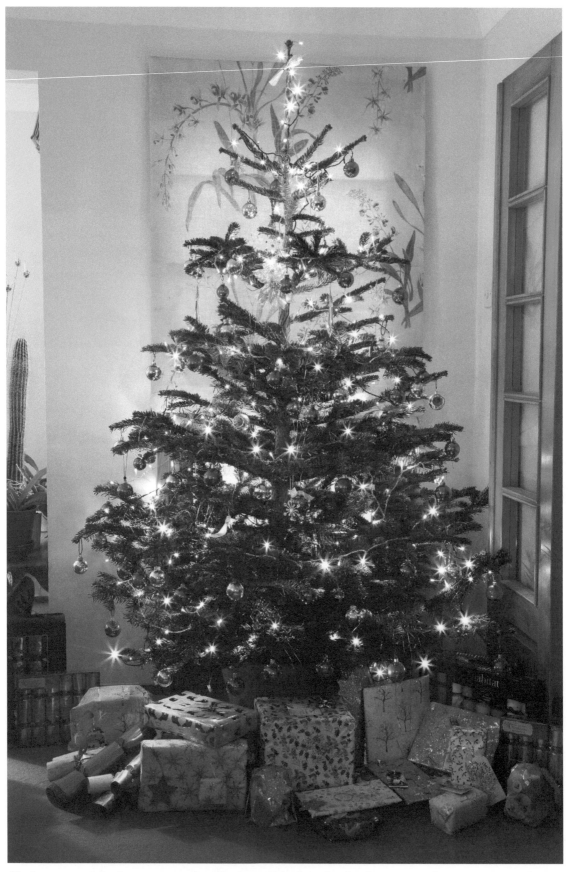

Christmas with the greater family but only for the lucky ones who weren't isolating

JANUARY 2022

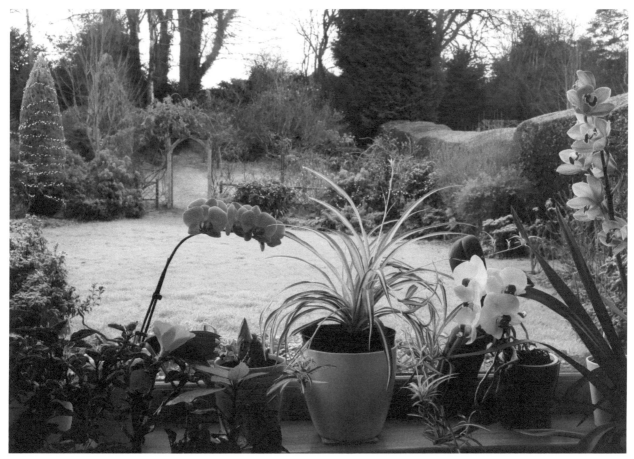

View of January garden through conservatory window.

Week 94.

January 1ˢᵗ 2022

It's the first day of a new year and there's optimism that 2022 will bring the end of the pandemic;
That mass immunity reduces hospitalization and death; Covid becomes manageable and endemic.

End of the pandemic would mean an era of sadness, restrictions and life of disruption would cease.
Alarming figures received on daily basis end, be relegated to the history books, such a happy release.

But for now they are all very real and relevant. Christmas and New Year are bound to swell numbers.
189,846 new cases recorded Friday, 11,918 in hospital and sadly 203 deaths; shockingly big figures.

In England last week one in 25 had Covid, 1 in 11 in London, I in 40 in Scotland, N. Ireland and Wales.
Omicron may be 75% less severe than Delta, but cases are 3 times higher. 90+% dominance prevails.

Nightingale surge hubs are to be set up in 8 hospitals in preparation for potential wave of Omicron.
Fitter patients in surge hubs will vacate hospital beds for seriously ill who need to be focused on.

UK has recorded a total of 148,421 deaths from Covid with 12,748,050 reported cases of infection.
With 5,448,536 deaths worldwide and 287,975,278 recorded cases, we all need time for reflection.

The New Year honours list put a smile on our faces. Those scientific characters were well rewarded.
Jenny Harries made a Dame. Chris Whitty and Johnathan Van-Tam, for their worthy work, knighted.

All three have been a trusted source of information on TV, presenting facts about Covid-19 disease.
They helped us to understand the spread, risk and nature of virus. Chris with his 'Next slide, please.'

PM, in year-end message, hailed 'heroic' vaccination effort. 'All adults have been offered a booster.'
He said UK's in an 'incomparably better position now than this time last year'. Situation's far better.

In England, there were no additional restrictions for New Year. We could celebrate as we pleased.
People urged to do lateral flow tests and party with caution but still fun with both hands was seized.

Scots advised not to travel to England to celebrate Hogmanay but stay at home to celebrate instead.
Closed nightclubs, social distancing, 3 household limit, knocked Hogmanay celebrations on the head.

Big Ben bongs were brought back, after nearly 4 years, to ring in 2022. Norm was back for Big Ben.
London's firework display was scaled back with no crowds. One day normality will return, but when?

MHRA have approved antiviral pill Paxlovid for use in UK. 2.75m courses of drug have been ordered. It's a protease inhibitor, blocks enzyme needed for the virus to multiply. It'll move recovery forward.

Fully vaccinated are now permitted to travel to Germany. Delhi imposes night curfew to slow spread. France allows UK citizens resident in EU countries to drive through as favour. Passage can go ahead.

It's been the mildest New Year on record. With no snow to adorn our gardens, we've used lights. Merryfield, Somerset recorded record high temperature New Year's Eve, 15.8C with no frosty nights.

It was farewell to 2021 at midnight singing Auld Lang Syne. We're really not sorry to see it through. Then, with fireworks on the River Thames, we welcomed in New Year. We have high hopes for 2022.

Week 95
January 8th 2022

Workforce absenteeism is causing massive disruption to life as Omicron variant continues to spread.
Businesses warned to expect 25% of staff to be absent in coming weeks are advised to look ahead.

Train timetables have been reduced as transport workforce depleted. Gatwick Express is suspended.
5,000 armed forces deployment to help in hospitals in medical and other capacities is expected.

ONS found 1 in 15 tested positive for Covid in UK last week creating a total of 3.7m people infected.
1 in 20 in Scotland and Wales, 1 in 25 N. Ireland, 1 in 10 London. Eye-watering but by Boris accepted.

PM announced there would be no further restrictions introduced in England in the next three weeks.
Said country could 'ride out' Omicron surge without further curbs. It is lack of disruption he seeks.

Saturday 146.390 new cases, 18,454 in hospital and 313 deaths. UK figures continue to proliferate.
150,057 total deaths within 28 days of positive test but 173,561 have Covid-19 on death certificate.

France recorded 335,000 new cases of Covid on 5 Jan. King and Queen of Sweden tested positive.
Italy is introducing compulsory vaccination for over 50s; infections unmanageable and excessive.

Yuzhou in China, a city of 1.2m, is in hard lockdown after three asymptomatic cases were identified.
 US recorded 1m positive Covid cases in 24 hours. Biden said it is a pandemic of the unvaccinated.

In Westminster, London, 4 in 10 haven't been vaccinated and it's the unvaccinated mostly in ICU.
But of the increasing number admitted to hospital, of those seriously ill there are relatively few.

UKHSA data shows 3 months after boosting, protection from serious disease is 90% for the over 65s.
But protection from mild symptomatic infection is short-lived. Drops to 30%, after 3 months it dives.

Schools returned this week. It is now mandatory for year 7 upwards to wear masks at school all day.
Advice is to open top windows. 7,000 air purifiers will be supplied to schools next month, they say.

New rules on travel testing are coming into force. No testing will be needed before departure to UK.
2-day test after arrival is lateral flow test, no longer PCR, but you'll need a 'fit to fly' test to go away.

ONS found 1.3m have long Covid. 892,000 contracted Covid 12 weeks ago, 500,000 one year earlier.
Common symptoms are extreme tiredness, shortness of breath, palpitations and brain fog or similar.

Anti-viral medication is being offered to vulnerable and immune-suppressed. It speeds up recovery.
Molnupiravir is already in use and Paxlovid, by Pfizer, will become available by the end of January.

NHS reported A & E exceptionally busy during lockdown with people trying to find a new activity.
5,300 admitted to hospital after falling from child playground attractions; 8 of them were over 90.

The days are getting longer and spring is only 2 months away. Hopefully, there is room for optimism.
Omicron wave should peak soon, we hope. Then we can embrace the future with eager enthusiasm.

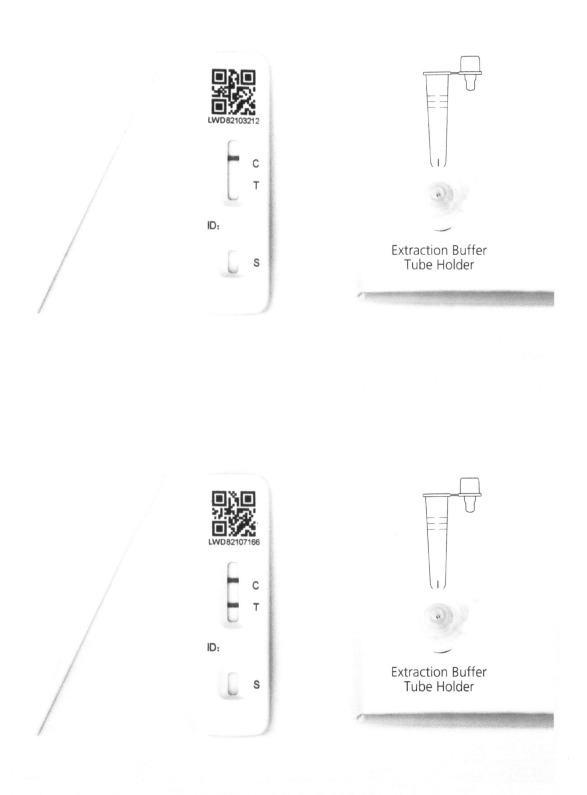

Top photograph: negative lateral flow test.
Below: positive lateral flow test (Antigen rapid test).

Covid – 19 Timeline

2019

December   Outbreak of a novel virus in Wuhan China

2020

30th January   WHO declared Public Health Emergency of international concern

31st January   First UK cases

23rd March   UK national lockdown ordered

28th May   Test and Trace launched in England

5th November   Four-week lockdown ordered in England

8th December   Vaccine programme began

2021

4th January   New lockdown ordered in England

20th March   Half of UK adults have had one dose

10th July   Legal restrictions end in England

24th November   South Africa reported Omicron variant to WHO

26th November   First cases of Omicron found in UK

31st December   All adults have been offered a Pfizer booster jab

Politicians, scientists and others mentioned in 'Covid Chronicles in Rhyme'.

Andy Burnham	Mayor of Greater London from 2017
Angela Merkel	Chancellor of Germany from 2005
Boris Johnson	Prime Minister of UK from July 2019
Captain Tom Moore	Raised money for charity in 2020 as he approached his 100th birthday
Dame Sarah Gilbert	Prof Sarah Gilbert, Oxford, Project Leader for the Oxford-AstraZeneca vaccine
Dominic Cummings	Chief advisor to Prime Minister Boris Johnson July 2019–November 2020
Donald Trump	US President from 2017 - 2021
Dolly Parton	US country singer. Funded development of a vaccine giving million dollars
Dr Jenny Harries	Chief Executive of the UK Health Security Agency from April 2021. Deputy Chief Medical Officer for England June 2019–April 2021 Made a Dame in the 2022 New Year Honours list.
Emmanuel Macron	President of France from 14th May 2017
Gavin Williams	Secretary of State for Education 2019 -2020
Grant Shapps	Secretary of State for Transport of the United Kingdom from 2019
Jeremy Corbyn	Leader of Labour Party and Leader of the Opposition from 2015–2020
Joe Biden	US President from 2021
Laura Kuenssberg	Political Editor for BBC from July 2015
Lord Deighton	Appointed 'PPE tsar' by Boris Johnson 19 April 2020, in charge PPE supplies
Mark Drakeford	First Minister of Wales and Leader of Welsh Labour party since 2018
Matt Hancock	Secretary of State for Health and Care 2018 – June 2021
Nicola Sturgeon	First Minister of Scotland and Leader of the Scottish National Party from 2014
Prof Patrick Valence	Chief Scientific Adviser to the UK Government from 2018
Prof Chris Whitty	Chief Medical Officer for England and Chief Medical Advisor from 2019 Knighted in 2022 New Year Honours list
Prof Jonathan Van-Tam	Deputy Chief Medical Officer for England from October 2017 Knighted in 2022 New Year Honours list
Prof Sharon Peacock	Professor of Public Health and Microbiology in Department of Medicine at the University of Cambridge
Rishi Sunak	Chancellor of Exchequer of UK from 2020

Sadiq Khan	Mayor of London from 2016
Sajid Javid	Secretary of State for Health and Care from June 2021
Sir Kier Starmer	Leader of Labour Party and Leader of the Opposition from April 2020
Queen Elizabeth II	Queen of the UK and 15 Commonwealth Countries Reference in text: Our Queen, Monarch

Abbreviations used in text

AC	After Covid (author's abbreviation invention)
A & E	Accident and Emergency
AGILE	Association of Geographic Information Laboratories of Europe.
AZ	Oxford/AstraZeneca vaccine
BAME	Black, Asian and Minority Ethnic
BA	British Airways
B & B	Bed and breakfast
BBC	British Broadcasting Corporation
BC	Before Covid (author's abbreviation invention)
BMI	Body mass index
CPAP	Continuous positive airway pressure. Pressurized air delivered through a mask
CVP	Covid-19 vaccine programme
EU	European Union
FDA	Food and Drug Administration (US)
FFP	Filtering facepiece
FFP1	Mask that traps larger dirt particles
FFP2	Mask that traps finer dust particles and aerosols (Effective for Covid protection)
FFP3	Most effective protector against bacteria and viruses.
FM	First Minister
G7	Group of Seven (Organization of the world's largest economies)
GCSE	General Certificate of Secondary Education
GM-CSF	Cytokine - Granulocyte-Macrophage Colony-Stimulating Factor.
GP	General Practitioner
ICU	Intensive care unit
JVCI	Joint Committee on Vaccination and Immunisation.
LBC	London Broadcasting Company
LFT	Lateral flower test or antigen test.
N95	Close-fitting disposable particle filtering mask
NASA	National Aeronautics and Space Administration
NIHP	National Institute for Health Policy
NE	North East

NHS	National Health Service
NHSX	National Health Service test and trace app
NIAID	National Institute of Allergy and Infectious Diseases
NW	North West
ONS	Office of National Statistics
PCR	Polymerase chain reaction test. Technique which amplifies DNA from virus sample
PHE	Public Health England
PM	Prime Minister
P & O	Pacific and Orient (passenger shipping line)
PPE	Personal protection equipment
REACT	Real-time Assessment of Community Transmission
RBD	Receptor-binding domain. Key part of virus allowing it to gain entry into cells
RNA/mRNA	Ribonucleic Acid. Ribonucleic Acid Messenger
R number	Reproduction number (Used to gauge how many one infected person infects)
SARS-CoV-2	Severe acute respiratory syndrome coronavirus 2. Coronavirus causing Covid-19
SE	South East
SNP	Scottish National Party
T2	Heathrow Terminal 2
T4	Tier 4
T5	Heathrow Terminal 5
TV	Television
UAE	United Arab Emirates
UN	United Nations
UK	United Kingdom
UKHSA	United Kingdom Health Security Agency
US	United States of America
VE Day	Victory in Europe
VP	Vice President of USA
WC	With Covid (author's abbreviation invention)
WHO	World Health Organization